Narrative Approaches in Play with Children

by the same author

The Story So Far
Play Therapy Narratives
Edited by Ann Cattanach
ISBN 978 1 84310 063 8

Process in the Arts Therapies
Edited by Ann Cattanach
ISBN 978 1 85302 625 6

Children's Stories in Play Therapy
Ann Cattanach
ISBN 978 1 85302 362 0

Play Therapy
Where the Sky Meets the Underworld
Ann Cattanach
ISBN 978 1 85302 211 1

Play Therapy with Abused Children
Ann Cattanach
ISBN 978 1 85302 193 0

of related interest

'If You Turned into a Monster'
Transformation through Play: A Body-Centred Approach
to Play Therapy
Dennis McCarthy
Foreword by Richmond K. Greene
ISBN 978 1 84310 529 9

Replays
Using Play to Enhance Emotional and Behavioral Development
for Children with Autism Spectrum Disorders
Karen Levine and Naomi Chedd
ISBN 978 1 84310 832 0

Drama Therapy and Storymaking in Special Education
Paula Crimmens
ISBN 978 1 84310 291 5

Narrative Approaches in Play with Children

Ann Cattanach

Jessica Kingsley Publishers
London and Philadelphia

First published in 2008
by Jessica Kingsley Publishers
116 Pentonville Road
London N1 9JB, UK
and
400 Market Street, Suite 400
Philadelphia, PA 19106, USA

www.jkp.com

Copyright © Ann Cattanach 2008
Printed digitally since 2010

Library of Congress Cataloging in Publication Data
A CIP catalog record for this book is available from the Library of Congress

British Library Cataloguing in Publication Data
A CIP catalogue record for this book is available from the British Library

ISBN 978 1 84310 588 6

Contents

Introduction
What is Narrative Play?

A Song

Tell me a story
Tell me a story
Tell me a story before I go to bed
Tell me about the bumble bees
Tell me about your clarty knees
Tell me a story before I go to bed.

The stories we tell about ourselves and our communities

This is a book about stories created in imaginary play and the way they impact upon our lives. From childhood we learn about ourselves from the stories other people tell us and the stories we tell about ourselves. From these stories we begin to form our identity and a sense of self. Some of these stories make us proud and strong in the sense of who we are, but this is not always so.

Dominant stories

Some dominant stories told about us in our families or the wider community can make us feel bad and worthless. I remember the torment of maths lessons at school because the teacher constantly mocked me, even imitating the way I walked and sat. Her story about me was that I was stupid. I lost confidence in myself and my ability to solve any maths problem. 'Stupid at maths' became part of my story about myself which I told to myself and others in my world. This concept was never tested because I was too afraid to find out if I had any ability or not.

Listening to children

The key to helping children develop a strong sense of self through stories and narratives in play is the relationship between child and adult as they play together. The adult may be the child's carer, parent or professional worker but in all situations the child and adult co-construct together. The child plays and the adult listens with empathy and perhaps asks questions to clarify the child's intentions. In this relationship some of the unhelpful dominant stories which the child has processed and which emerge in imaginative play can be evaluated and changes can be made. There is an equality in this relationship and it is the quality which the adult listener brings which can determine the nature of the interchanges in the play. So the adults must value play not only for the child but also as a life-enhancing process in their relationship.

Stories children tell and stories adults tell children

Family stories

From the age of two most children develop pretend play and use this process to make sense of their world and culture. The lives of some children in families are fraught with danger and fear and this will be represented in their pretend play. Mary, aged four, invented the following story which in many ways mimicked her reality world and the desire that environment had created in her to destroy everything and everyone to be free from pain and fear.

> Once upon a time there was a wicked witch and a wicked
> dragon.
> They lived together.
> They put the birdie in the cage.
> They hurt the birdie and hit it.
> They drank a lot.
> They hurt the dog and the baby.
> The wicked witch is dead.
> Mary killed her.
> She put the animals in the cage and shot the animals.
> They are all dead.

Stories about where we live

We tell stories about the places we live, our town, village or city and the country we inhabit; where we came from and where we live now. Jim was a young boy I worked with many years ago, helping him move from a small residential home into an adoptive family. His play was always through role taking with themes of Jack-the-lad ducking and diving and searching for adult approval.

As a very young child he had lived in London with his mother, who struggled with mental health problems. Jim learned to manage his life by befriending people on the street by his home. There were many shops there and Jim moved around the street keeping warm in shops and being fed by the fish and chip man. The school traffic warden befriended him and he was supported in this environment.

When the time came to leave the children's home and live in a family, we went to say goodbye to all his friends on the street. The fish and chip man and his family had looked out for Jim, kept him safe, and sent him home well fed. We went down the street saying goodbye to his friends. He said he would miss the bustle of city life where he had learnt his social skills, who to trust, and the values of that wider community. He was lucky to find a broader family who kept him safe until he moved to the children's home. He also enjoyed the smell of the street, the look of the buildings and remembered the warm nooks and crannies where he had huddled to keep himself warm after school before he went back home. He said he would remember the street for ever as it was part of the story of his life, but now he had his own family.

Cultural stories

Then there are the cultural stories told to us about our place in the family and the wider community. If the family culture is one of violence, cruelty or demeaning women then the child learns this culture and these stories enter their perception of their world. I remember a father who gave his children names which created the initials GBH and ABH, reinforcing the family view that violence was their cultural norm.

These inner representations of their world emerge in the imaginary stories children tell in play. Ken was a 13-year-old boy who had lived in a family where drug addiction led to violent encounters with dealers. He told the following story using small figures in slime to depict the fear.

The Lake of Blood and Guts Island

The lake of blood and guts was in a hot country.
It was a horrible place and tons and tons of creatures lived there.
They were all evil, nobody good.
They ate humans especially children.
They lived in a messy pile biting each other and fighting.
They were druggies, drunkards, did everything I've mentioned and swam about in the blood and the guts.
Outside of the lake was a pile of blue shit which was being eaten by a lizard.
He eated shit a lot.
He ate the shit then shat the shit.
He was a horrible lizard and the others called him a pile of shit.
Everybody who lived there on this huge pile liked it because they didn't have anything else and didn't want to go anywhere else not ever.
They all shit a lot.
It was a chaotic life for everybody.

If this is Ken's inner representation of the world then he has no place of safety or any adults to keep him secure. In reality and in his play world Ken didn't trust adults to care for him because this had never happened. He couldn't represent what he didn't know.

Cultural stories which define ethnicity are very important to families and the wider community to help structure a group identity. This can be especially important to communities who have been displaced and are trying to make a new home for themselves in an unfamiliar environment with different rules and customs.

I sometimes tell the story of *The Three Brothers* to families or children who struggle with two cultures. This is a story of a life split in two where the hero returns to his familiar home. This can be an expression of the longing for home which can be the dream of those who are displaced.

The Three Brothers

There were once three brothers who belonged to the Arapaho Indian tribe. They were all good hunters but the youngest brother always had the best luck hunting. The older brothers became very jealous of him.

'Let us kill Little Eagle,' said the eldest brother, 'and then the other hunters will stop jeering at us.' So Wild Bear the eldest and Red Horse the middle brother decided to take Little Eagle hunting then lose him in the forest so far away from home that he wouldn't be able to find his way back.

So when the tribe were out hunting the three brothers went off together as usual. The two wicked brothers pushed further and further, drawing Little Eagle away from the rest of the tribe. Suddenly, when Little Eagle was examining the animal tracks the two wicked brothers attacked him from behind and he fell senseless to the ground. But as they were about to kill him they heard the cries of the other hunters and they hurried off in their direction to make it appear that nothing had happened. They told the rest of the tribe that Little Eagle had gone off to track some wonderful animal and would rejoin them later.

Little Eagle lay in the bushes all night because his brothers had given him such a terrible beating.

One of the Enchanted Beings who guide the affairs of men found him and brought him back to consciousness. But he was still badly injured and could not see, so the Enchanted Being guided him to the tents of some friendly Indians.

These Indians were blood brothers of the Arapaho and he spent many months with them. His wounds healed but he still did not remember what had happened. He did not know his name or who he was. So he stayed with his new friends and was accepted by the old chief who felt sorry for him. Little Eagle became known as Two Persons: the man he had been and forgotten and the man he was now.

In time Two Persons became a great hunter and was admired by the young men of his adopted tribe. They weren't jealous, as his brothers had been. Sometimes Two Persons did wonder who he was. He knew he was an Arapaho because of the way the beads were sewn on his shirt, his leggings and the small pouch he wore on his belt.

The chief had a daughter called Blue Stone and she fell in love with Two Persons but she knew that it was impossible for him to ask her hand in marriage because he was a nameless man with no tent of his own.

Two Persons brought food for the tribe and could eat with the men with no shame, but although he loved Blue Stone he felt powerless to approach her.

One night the Enchanted Being came to him in a dream and told him of his past. He told him his name and where he was born and what his brothers had done to him. He said it was time for Little Eagle to return to his tribe but first he must ask for the hand of Blue Stone and take her back with him as his wife. He said that his brothers no longer wanted to kill him. The Enchanted Being gave Little Eagle instructions for the journey.

Next day Little Eagle went to the old chief and told him the whole story. He asked for Blue Stone to be his wife if she were willing. The chief knew his daughter's mind and agreed. So Little Eagle took Blue Stone's hand and they went to collect a few herbs as the Enchanted Being had instructed in the dream.

Little Eagle's home was far away and the journey took a long time. When they got to the place where he had been born they found that the people in his tribe were stricken by a mysterious illness. It was called the spotted sickness and was in fact smallpox brought by some of the first white men to come to their land.

Little Eagle and his wife knew what they must do. They boiled the herbs they had brought and made an infusion which they gave to the sick. Some lived and some died but the medicine helped many to recover.

Little Eagle's two brothers Wild Bear and Red Horse were changed in their appearance by the smallpox but the medicine helped to save their lives. The brothers begged Little Eagle to forgive them for their cruelty to him in the past. They knew he had saved their lives with the medicine he had brought.

Little Eagle forgave them and when they were well and strong again they went out hunting together. The two brothers rejoiced that Little Eagle was alive and they hadn't killed him.

The Enchanted Being looked after Little Eagle and preserved his life so he became a great hunter honoured by the tribe and loved forever by his wife Blue Stone.

We tell our own stories and from childhood hear the fictional stories of our own and other people's cultures. This can lead to a greater understanding of ourselves and the wider world. And for children it is often comforting to know that other people have similar experiences to their own. Children's imaginative stories and narratives merge with other cultural stories to form part of an autobiography which helps to define their place in the world.

Learning about ourselves through cultural stories

We all tell our stories in different ways, so to begin here is a selection of stories demonstrating a variety of views of the world. Sharing cultural stories helps children understand that their views are shared by others and that many struggles have a universal quality. To generalize a difficulty can be a comfort and children often accept what is in a story rather than a personal challenge about their behaviour.

Accepting advice

This first story is an English folk tale about a girl who finds it difficult to accept advice, fearing humiliation, but eventually learns to listen.

The Girl Who Fetched Water in a Riddle *

One day a little girl took a riddle to a well to fetch some water, but the water ran out of the riddle as fast as she poured it in. Two little robins who were sitting on a hedge close by watched her as they twittered their songs. The birds made such a noise that the girl thought they were laughing at her, so she said, 'Silly robins, how can I take water in a riddle?'

The robins said,

> Stuff your riddle with moss,
> And daub it with clay,
> And carry your water
> Right away.

---

* A riddle is a large sieve used in the garden.

But the little girl said, 'I shan't, you ugly birds,' and dipped her riddle into the well again. The water ran out of the riddle again, but the third time the little girl did as the robins had told her, when the riddle held the water and the robins were pleased.

Many children who have had to be a parent to their parents find it difficult to ask and receive help and are very resistant to offers of advice or loss of control. Other children carry labels of disability and want to show they can manage, so again resist. This little story helps them understand that they are not the only children who have this struggle.

Risk taking

This great British tale of Tommy Grimes is a story for those boys who are risk takers, not thinking of consequences and learning only by direct experience.

Mr Miacca

Tommy Grimes was sometimes a good boy and sometimes a bad boy, and when he was a bad boy he was a very bad boy.

Now his mother used to say to him, 'Tommy, Tommy be a good boy and don't go out on the street or else Mr Miacca will take you.'

But still when he was a bad boy he would go out on the street and one day, sure enough, he had scarcely got round the corner when Mr Miacca did catch him and popped him into a bag upside down and took him off to his house.

When Mr Miacca got Tommy inside he pulled him out of the bag and set him down and felt his arms and legs. 'You're rather tough,' said he, 'but you're all I've got for supper and you'll not taste bad boiled. But body of me I've forgotten the herbs and it's bitter you'll taste without herbs. Sally, here I say Sally,' and he called Mrs Miacca.

So Mrs Miacca came into the room and said, 'What do you want my dear?'

'Here a little boy for supper and I've forgotten the herbs. Mind him while I go for them.'

'All right my love,' says Mrs Miacca and off he goes.

Then Tommy Grimes said to Mrs Miacca, 'Does Mr Miacca always have little boys for supper?'

'Mostly, my dear,' says Mrs Miacca, 'if little boys are bad enough to get in his way.'

'And don't you have anything else but boy meat? No pudding?'

'Ah, I love pudding,' says Mrs Miacca, 'but it's not often the likes of me gets pudding.'

'Why my mother is making a pudding this very day,' says Tommy, 'and I'm sure she'll give you some if I ask her. Shall I run and get some?'

'Now that's a very thoughtful boy,' says Mrs Miacca, 'only don't be long and be sure to be back for supper.'

So off Tommy peltered and right glad he was to get off so cheap and for many a long day he was as good as good could be and he never went round the corner of the street.

But he couldn't always be good and one day he went round the corner and, as luck would have it, he hadn't scarcely gone round it when Mr Miacca grabbed him up, popped him in his bag and took him home.

When he got there Mr Miacca dropped him out and when he saw him he said, 'Ah, you're the youngster who tricked me and my missus leaving us without any supper. Well you shan't do it again. I'll watch over you myself. Here get under the sofa and I'll set on it and watch the pot boil for you.'

So poor Tommy Grimes had to creep under the sofa and Mr Miacca sat on it and waited for the pot to boil.

And they waited and waited and waited and still the pot didn't boil till at last Mr Miacca got tired of waiting and he said, 'Here you under there I'm not going to wait any longer; put out your leg and I'll stop you giving us the slip.'

So Tommy put out a leg, and Mr Miacca got a chopper and chopped it off and put it in the pot.

Suddenly he calls out, 'Sally, my dear Sally,' and nobody answered.

So he went into the next room to look out for Mrs Miacca and while he was there Tommy Grimes crept from under the sofa and ran out of the door.

For it was the leg of the sofa that he had put out.

So Tommy Grimes ran home, and he never went round the corner again till he was old enough to go alone.

The story is funny but has that element of fear and menace which has shock value. Mr Miacca eats children, but Tommy doesn't think of consequences, so one contact with Mr Miacca doesn't teach Tommy to avoid danger and on the second visit he nearly gets chopped up for the pot. Finally he learns. And the sane advice is to wait until you are old and wise enough to venture 'round the corner'.

People and their places

Stories often include mythical creatures evolved from the place and the history of the people who live there. Johnny Croy is a mermaid story originally from Orkney. Mermaids, seals who change into people, people who change into sea creatures, all are themes from sea and fishing environments. When times are difficult inhabitants often leave their communities and this is reflected in the stories of humans who go to live with the merfolk and merfolk who are forced to live on the land.

Johnny Croy and the Mermaid

This is the story my grandmother told me about my parents before she died.

In those days before I was born my grandmother lived by the sea with my father, Johnny Croy, who was a fisherman. Grandmother said he was a handsome, smart kind of man and all the girls fancied him, but he couldn't find anyone to love so he kept on fishing and swaggering about the beach and flirting with the visitors but making no commitments to anyone but himself and my grandmother, his mother.

Some fishermen teased him, calling him Sharkie because of his skill at capturing fish and girls, especially those summer girls who came on their holidays looking for romance. He was good at romancing the girls but for himself he seemed to be waiting for some great adventure, some magical person who would change his life. And one winter's day, when the visitors had gone and the beach was quiet, it happened.

He was mending his lobster pots and just enjoying the sea and the sand and the smell of the willow stems as he made his repairs.

And then he saw her, the most fragile golden haired creature sitting on the rocks combing her hair with the most exquisite comb made of gold, encrusted with rubies and sapphires.

He said it was the gold of the hair and the movement of the comb that took his breath away. Gold on gold and he wanted both.

The creature was singing, the voice was exquisite. The song described with such sweetness the longing and desire that was love.

He was mesmerized, and in that moment of seeing the mermaid he knew he must win her for his wife. He crept behind the rocks on the beach then moved down the shore until he was between her and the sea. He crept up behind her, put his arms around her waist. She turned round to face him and he kissed her on the mouth. His arms became entangled in her hair which he stroked as he kissed her again and again. She was shocked and angry. She lifted her silver petticoats and struck him very hard with her tail. He was flattened by the blow and rolled in agony on the beach.

The mermaid slid from the rocks into the sea and Johnny Croy, still winded by the blow from her tail, crawled down the sand in pursuit. The mermaid floated in the water and stared at Johnny Croy. She was burning with anger but on seeing his beauty her anger became tempered with a kind of passion for the man.

They stared at one another.

Johnny got to his feet and as he pulled himself up he saw something glistening in the sand. It was the mermaid's comb. It must have fallen from her hair when he kissed her. Johnny knew that the possession of the mermaid's comb gave him power over her.

She knew that in her kingdom a mermaid without her comb becomes a creature to be ridiculed and shamed. The loss of her comb meant the loss of her honour and her status in the sea kingdom. She pleaded with Johnny Croy. 'Please give me back my comb.'

But Johnny was overcome by his love for her. 'Come and live with me. I have a fine house, land, cattle and I am skilled at fishing.'

She refused. 'I could never live on the land. The rain, snow, mists are not like the sea world. And your fires keep you warm but would destroy my skin. I would shrivel in such a place. Why don't you come and live in my world and be my merrow? You understand the sea and have fished and sailed all your life. Life under the sea is even more exotic. We have gold and jewels and fine palaces and cattle, and gardens. Be my merrow. The Fin Folk will take to you.'

They both argued for their own territory but could not convince the other.

The more they spoke to each other the more their desire grew, but love of their own kind was stronger and in the end the mermaid left Johnny Croy alone on the beach holding her golden comb. As she swam away from him she sang another song of loss for her love and her comb. Johnny walked home with her sweet voice ringing in his ears.

He told his mother, my grandmother, about his meeting and showed her the comb. She was a wise old woman renowned in that part as a walker between worlds so she knew that he was speaking the truth.

She berated her son for his foolishness. 'Just like a man to fall in love with one from another world when there are plenty here who would love you. Men are all the same. Well if I can't persuade you to let her be, then keep her golden comb, which is her dearest treasure, and then you will have power over her. But my advice is to throw the comb back into the sea and leave her in peace to find her own merrow.'

Grandmother knew he would not listen to her and would pursue his heart's desire. She felt love for him and sadness because she knew that such passion for one from the sea could only bring misfortune and sorrow for them all.

Johnny was obsessed by his passion for the mermaid. He wondered what would happen if he followed her into the sea. He remembered the story of the seal folk. Would he be like the Great Silkie of Skule Skerrie?

> I am a man upon the land,
> And I am a Silkie in the sea,
> And when I'm far and far from land,
> My dwelling is in Skule Skerrie.

If he went with the mermaid, would he become a merrow with a fish's tail?

Merrows were reputed to be vicious creatures, not seductive like the mermaids. Would he stay with his human form and drown or would he be able to inhabit a fish form so he could survive under the sea and live like the Great Silkie?

He felt such passion for the mermaid and he knew that somehow they must live together somewhere. He called her My Lovely Gem and waited for her to come to him again as he knew she must.

One night as he drifted in and out of sleep, he thought he heard the magical singing of the mermaid. He sat up with a start and saw her sitting by the window of his room. He tried once again to persuade her to come and live with him in his beautiful house but she shook her head.

'I'll make a bargain with you,' she said. 'I'll live here with you for seven years but at the end of that time you and all that's mine must come and live with me under the sea.'

Johnny thought that was a fair bargain so he agreed and he and My Lovely Gem were married and lived happily together for seven years. During that time they produced seven children. And that is where I enter the story.

I was a small baby, the seventh child.

The seven years had come to an end and it was time for the family to leave and live in the sea kingdom. Johnny, my father, kept his side of the bargain and the family prepared to embark in his boat and leave.

But the night before departure I was left with my grandmother as my father and mother had a lot to arrange. Grandmother was about to lose all her family. It was intolerable.

She was a wise woman and knew fairy lore. She was determined not to lose us all so she took some wire and made a thin iron cross, heated it on the fire and branded me with the cross on my backside.

She said that I screamed the house down.

And even now, I sometimes wake screaming at night and feel a burning pain all over my body and then I remember my mother holding me, loving me, wanting me and then the despair of my grandmother who knew she was to be abandoned.

The next day the boat was ready and many of my mother's fin folk came to help. My brothers and sisters were carried to the boat. They were excited, wanting to start their new adventure.

My mother and father came down from the big house. Mother came to get me from grandmother's house but when she tried to lift me a burning pain shot through her arms and she couldn't prise me from the cradle.

The power and the magic of that time are strong even now. I feel her arms touching me holding me, and her screams as she too felt the burn of the brand paralysing her fingers, arms and body until she could hold me no longer. Both of us branded, shamed, lost to each other forever.

My mother had to leave me behind.

Grandmother had got me, I was her possession now, but she cried for the rest of her family lost to her forever.

The boat sailed away and my mother sang a song of such loss and despair that it broke the hearts of all who heard it. 'Alas, alas for my bonny bairn, my beautiful boy who will live and die on the land.'

The boat disappeared into the mist with only the haunting sound of her song and they were never seen again.

Comic world views

One of my favourite artists is David Shrigley (2003). I like his mordant view of the world. He creates both drawings and texts. I use his texts with adolescents struggling towards a changed identity in an adult world.

I TRY TO PUSH MYSELF FORWARD
EVERY DAY

FIRST I FIND A STARTING POINT
AND I START THERE.
I SELECT A BOOK FROM THE
BIG TIT LIBRARY AND I SIT
READING IT. THEN I DO MY
CHORES WHICH ARE BORING.
THEN I ASK FOR A CUP OF
TEA AND THE GIRL SAYS WHAT
STRAIN OF TEA DO I WANT?
AND I SAY BUILDERS' TEA.
THEN SHE QUESTIONS ME
ABOUT THE INDELIBLE MARKS
ON MY CLOTHES AND I SAY
IT WASN'T ME AND SHE SAYS
THAT I AM THE ULTIMATE
TORMENT.

'I Try to Push Myself Forward Every Day' reproduced with permission from David Shrigley (2003) Who I Am and What I Want. *London: Redstone Press.*

What is narrative play?

Narrative play is a way of communicating with children using stories and narratives to share and make sense of life events. It is a collaborative approach where the adult helps the child order their experiences through the use of imaginative play processes.

Michael Frayn (2006) says that our mental life is interpretive all the time: we make our thoughts by having them, and mould our feelings by the way we feel them. Engel (1995) states that every story a child tells contributes to a self-portrait, which he or she can look at, refer to, think about and change, and this portrait can be used by others to develop an understanding of the storyteller. The stories we tell, whether they are about real or imagined events, convey our experience, our ideas, and a dimension of who we are.

The adult and child construct a space and a relationship together where the child can develop a personal and social identity by finding stories to tell about the self and the lived world of that self. The partnership agreement between child and adult gives meaning to the play as it happens. The stories created in this playing space may not be 'true' but will often be genuine and powerfully felt and expressed.

Social constructionist stance

This way of working uses themes developed in social construction theory. Burr and Butt (2000) state that post-modern thought proposes that we will never be able to penetrate 'the real' with our imperfect perceptions and constructions. But we are naturally sense-making beings who interpret events and confer meanings upon things. We experience an objective world out there that is revealed to us through our senses. And there is a split between that objective world and our subjective under-standing of it, and the world we experience lies somewhere between subject experience and objective world. What we experience is both made and found. So we are limited both by events in the world and by our constructions of those events. We might describe this as the 'lived' world. The perceived world is not a more or less perfect replica of objective reality: we manipulate that reality and we produce constructions that serve our purposes and help us in our projects.

Hermeneutic approach

This social constructionist view of the world is a hermeneutic approach. Hermeneutics is the activity of interpreting and explores how meaning is constructed through language discourse, story and narrative. In this form of analysis the world appears as we interpret it, and the search for meaning is ongoing. Knowledge is a socially interpreted event con-structed through relationships and conversation with others. Anderson and Goolishian (1992) state that a therapist working in a hermeneutic way lets the person's story unfold until a coherent theme or new meaning emerges from the dialogue. It is the therapist's curiosity to know more about what is being said – that is, how a client makes meaning – that engages the future or 'not-yet-said' narrative. Therapeutic conversation involves a mutual search for understanding in which the therapist and client talk 'with' not 'to' each other. This not-knowing hermeneutic stance is the therapist's expertise to support the child in finding their own meaning in understanding their own problem. This communication style can be used by any adult listening and playing with a child. The key to the relationship is the adult's capacity to listen and reflect with the child. Read and consider the West African Story of the Hungry Elephant.

The Story of the Hungry Elephant

Once there lived an elephant, and he said to himself, 'I am hungry.' He went along a path in the forest and came to a bamboo-palm standing in a swamp.

Roughly he tore down the palm. He saw a tender bud in one of its leaves, but as he took the bud from the leaf it fell into the water.

He hunted and hunted yet could not find it because he had stirred up the water and it blinded his eyes.

Then a frog spoke and said, 'Listen.'

The elephant did not hear, thrashing the water hard with his trunk.

The frog spoke again: 'Listen.'

The elephant heard this time, and stood perfectly still, curious.

Thereupon the water became clear so that he found the palm-bud and ate it.

The basis of narrative play is to explore the stories children present in play and facilitate an exchange of ideas and thoughts about the stories. This approach means that the relationship between child and adult is one of co-construction, sharing ideas and listening to each other to find the story which best supports the child in what they want to say. This is a hermeneutic stance because the adult's listening response is a continuous enquiry towards the material presented in a play session. This developing narrative always presents the adult with the next question. This is a 'not knowing' position; the adult's understanding is always developing.

The narrative focus

White (2005) lists a series of concepts which describe his key ideas of narrative as a therapy. He states that the primary focus of a narrative approach is people's expressions of their experiences of life. The narrative expressions of both adults and children act as interpretations and through these interpretations people give meaning to their experiences of life, which seem sensible to themselves and to others. He states that meaning does not pre-exist the interpretation of experience.

He considers that expressions are constitutive of life, the world that is lived through; they structure experience and inform future understanding. Expressions have a cultural context and are informed by the knowledge and practices of life that are culturally determined. The structure of narrative provides the principal frame of intelligibility for people in their day-to-day lives. It is through this frame that people link together the events of life in sequences that unfold through time according to specific themes.

A narrative therapy is about options for the telling and retelling of the preferred stories of people's lives, rendering the unique, the contradictory, the contingent and, at times, the aberrant events of people's lives significant as alternative presents. White and Epston (1990) make the assumption that individuals experience problems when the narratives in which they are storying their experience and/or in which they are having their experience storied by others do not sufficiently represent their lived experience and that in these circumstances there will be significant aspects of their lived experience that contradict these dominant narratives.

The functions of narratives and stories in play

If the adult uses a narrative approach in play with children, then the following functions can underpin and support the intervention.

1. Telling stories and playing stories can be a way of controlling our world and what happens to us in that world and for a child who lacks power it can be an enriching experience. For once the child can say, 'I'm the king of the castle, and you're the dirty rascal,' and not live the consequences in their reality world.

2. The use of narratives and stories in play can help children to make sense of their own lives and also to learn empathy through imagining how other characters in their stories might feel.

3. Working with stories and narrative play means that there is collaboration between child and adult where what happens in the sessions is co-constructed between the two.

4. This model is based on social construction theory and narrative therapy, which describe the development of identity as based on the stories we tell about ourselves and the stories others in our environment tell about us.

5. Some dominant stories we have about ourselves are not helpful and can lead to victimization. In play we can explore ways to shift and expand aspects of identity through exploring roles and ways of being in play knowing that we do not have to take all these experiments into our lived lives.

6. This approach also recognizes the fact that the developing child is part of an ecological system, not an isolated individual. We live in time and in a culture and this influences our way of seeing.

7. In this kind of collaboration the child plays with small toys and objects, or draws a picture or just makes marks on clay or slime, but as they do so they tell a story about what they are doing. The role of the adult is to listen, and perhaps ask questions about the story if required. Sometimes the adult can tell a story, which might be congruent with the play of the child or as a way to deepen the relationship by the shared experience of telling and listening.

Pretend play: the landscape of the imagination

Children develop their narratives and stories through pretend play and it is through entering this world that adult and child can develop a relationship which helps both participants in their understanding of their relationship, the world and their place in it. Pretend play requires the ability to transform objects and actions symbolically; it is developed through social dialogue and involves play with objects, role taking and improvisation.

Vygotsky (1978) considers that the criteria for distinguishing a child's play from other forms of activity is that in play a child creates an imaginary situation. He states that the creation of an imaginary situation is the first manifestation of the child's emancipation from situational constraints. The paradox of play is that the child operates with an alienated meaning in a real situation. Macy was longing for a family. Her stories were about this imaginary family who might in the future become her real family. In play they were shadowy figures or snow people who melted into thin air.

> So I was playing with Macy in her foster home. Macy made a sofa out of Play Doh. It had pink and blue pillows. I asked her who is going to sit on the sofa.
>
> 'Nobody, it is just there,' said Macy. 'There is a white snowman like a cushion on the sofa. Not a real snowman, it would just melt. It is a teddy snowman. The baby is sitting between two baby snowmen. They look after the baby.'
>
> I ask if the baby has a mum. Macy replies: 'Her old mum is dead but she has a new mum.'
>
> I ask if the mum has a name. Macy says: 'Mum has no name. The baby just calls her mum. The baby's name is Tom Tom.'

In reality Macy is waiting for a new family and has been in care for over two years. In play she is emancipated from that situation so she structures her story in a way which makes sense. Macy enjoys the experience and likes my questions, which help her develop her play story to her own satisfaction.

Engel (1995) holds that every story a child tells, acts out through play or writes contributes to a self-portrait…a portrait others can use to develop an understanding of the storyteller. And this expands his or her world. She considers that stories are both a product of a developmental process and a vehicle through which development takes place.

Vygotsky (1978) says that there is great pleasure for the child in the act of playing an imaginary story but in order to achieve the greatest pleasure and satisfaction the child must learn and keep the rules. So Macy and I have rules about playing together and as she structures her play and stories she is learning the rules of sequencing and coherence to make a story which satisfies her. In play, action is subordinated to meaning but in real life action dominates meaning. In her reality world, when Macy visits her birth family the environment is chaotic and she gets lost in the crowd. In her play world adults seem to be represented as snowmen who disappear and melt so are little comfort for the baby. Although the baby has a mum she is invisible, not yet realized, which is a reflection of her reality world. In her play the baby and teddy are the only solid characters, all the others are prone to disappear.

Children tell stories not only to represent experience as they know it to be but they also tell stories to represent experience as they would like it to be. The imaginative control you gain over the world by being able to decide, at least symbolically, who does what to whom and what things look like and sound like is itself a vital component of human experience.

Petra is 14, living in a small and loving children's home where she feels safe and contained. She has serious attachment issues with her birth family. She drew a heart and told this story:

> There was once a heart which belonged to no one.
> No one loved it and it floated in space like a loner.
> This heart had never belonged to anyone neither male nor female
> And it was broken.
> It had an arrow piercing the flesh, no blood, just a purple heart.
> And in the end it was exploded by an Iraqi bomb
> And spattered into a thousand and one pieces.
> It might possibly be put together again.
> But if it falls into another person it will be born again
> And the person with the purple heart
> Will be happy and live forever.
> The End.

This tentative expression of hope can be contained within a story, which is the safe place to express such desires because it does not have to be proved in the lived world.

The development of pretend play

Harris (2000) suggests that two-year-olds understand some of the essential ingredients of drama and fiction. They recognize episodes that are not to be construed as events in the real world but as events occurring within a make-believe framework. The episodes and events that are represented in the course of pretend play are fictional rather than real. It is an initial exploration of possible worlds.

Dunn (1993) states that babies play an active part in interactional games like peek-a-boo and later hide and seek, enjoying the give and take of the play. She defines this play as two or more individuals working towards a mutual goal, with alternation of turns and repetition of actions. She found that in the years between early infancy and nursery school babies as young as eight months are able to respond to the playful moods of their siblings, frequently imitating their actions. At 18 months the child is actively imitating their older siblings in pretend play, co-operating and imitating sequences of actions. The ability of children to co-operate in pretend play is one of the most striking features of the period between infancy and school.

Dunn's research also indicates that, during the second and third years, children can not only take one role in a joint game with siblings but were also able to reverse roles. The child begins this role-play at the sibling's suggestion but by the end of the second year the youngest child is able to take the initiative. This pretend play involves the capacity of the child to share a pretend framework with another person, to co-ordinate pretend actions, to be able to act as another person or thing and also to mutually explore social roles and rules.

Corsaro (1997) describes spontaneous fantasy play among younger three- and four-year-old children in an Italian pre-school setting. He states that the play often involved children becoming animals or imaginary characters like monsters, fairies or princesses through the manipulation of toy figures or physical embodiment. Children created and shared pretend routines with particular rules governing the nature of the play and the rights and obligations of players in the very course of the play activities. The play is highly improvisational and is often guided indirectly by underlying themes ('danger–rescue', 'lost–found', 'death–rebirth').

So play and storytelling are the basis of our learning about the world and our place in it, and woe betide those who won't share!

Why Everyone Should be Able to Tell a Story (A Scottish Story)

Once there was a Uist man who was travelling home. He had to come by the Isle of Skye, crossing the sea from Dunvegan to Lochmaddy. This man had been away working the harvest on the mainland

He was walking through Skye on his way home and at nightfall he came to a house and thought he would stay there till morning. He went in and was made welcome by the man of the house.

His host asked him if he had any stories or tales to tell. He replied that he had never known any.

'It's very strange that you can't tell a story,' said his host. 'I'm sure you've heard plenty.'

'I can't remember one,' said the Uist man.

His host himself was telling stories all night until it was time to go to bed.

When they went to bed the Uist man was given the closet inside the front door to sleep in. What was there hanging in the closet was the carcass of a sheep. The Uist man hadn't been long in bed when he heard the door being opened. Two men came in and took away the sheep. The Uist man said to himself that it would be very unfortunate for him if he let the two fellows take the sheep away, for the people of the house would think that he had stolen it. He went after the thieves.

After a time one of the thieves noticed him. He said to the other thief, 'Look at that fellow coming after us to betray us. Let's go back and catch him and do away with him.'

They turned back and the Uist man made off as fast as he could to get back to the house. But they got between him and the house.

The Uist man kept going until he heard the sound of a big river. Then he made for the river.

In his panic he went into the river and the stream took him away. He was likely to be drowned. But he got a hold of a branch of a tree that was growing on the bank of the river. And he clung onto it. He was too frightened to move.

He heard the two men going back and forth along the banks of the river. They were throwing stones wherever the trees cast their shade. And the stones were going past him. He stayed there until dawn. It was a frosty night.

When he tried to get out of the river he couldn't do it. He tried to shout but he couldn't shout either. At last he managed to utter one shout and he made a leap.

He woke up and found himself on the floor beside the bed, holding onto the bedclothes with both hands. His host had been casting spells on him during the night.

In the morning when they were at breakfast his host said, 'Well, I'm sure that wherever you are tonight you'll have a story to tell though you hadn't one last night. That's what happens to a man who couldn't tell a story. Everyone should be able to tell a tale or a story to help pass the night.'

CHAPTER 1

The Therapeutic Relationship
Thinking about Children

The social construction of childhood

It is important for adults who want to make supportive relationships with children to examine their own constructions of childhood and how that might impact on their relationship with the children they are trying to nurture and support.

In *The Invention of Childhood* (2006) Cunningham says that in the twenty-first century we don't all agree on when childhood begins and we certainly don't agree on when it ends. Likewise the contents of childhood are variable. We know what we don't like about childhood and children in the present – children who are obese, children who terrorize their neighbourhood, and children who bully other children. We also worry about children who seem to be in danger from the adult world, children who grow up too fast, the rising rate of mental illness among children, the one in twelve British children who self-harm. But turn the question round and ask how positively we would like to see childhood and we stumble. Cunningham suggests that some of our confusion is because we are heirs to so many conflicting views from the past, so many different inventions of childhood.

He discusses how we don't agree when childhood begins and ends. There are markers for beginnings like conception, birth, some point beyond babyhood and endings like puberty, when we leave school, when we leave home. We have no ceremonies or rituals, as in some societies, for the end of childhood. And the word 'child' is used in many different senses. For example, we are always the children of our parents and this continues throughout our lives.

In the United Nations Children's Fund (UNICEF) report 'An Overview of Child Well-being in Rich Countries' (2007) child well-being was measured and compared in 21 nations under six different headings or dimensions: material well-being, health and safety, education, peer and family relationships, behaviours and risks, and young people's own subjective sense of well-being. The main findings were that the Netherlands heads the table of overall child well-being, ranking in the top ten for all six dimensions, while the United Kingdom and the United States find themselves in the bottom third of the rankings for five of the six dimensions reviewed. There was no obvious relationship between levels of child well-being and gross domestic product (GDP) per capita. The report concludes that all families in Organisation for Economic Development and Cooperation (OECD) countries today are aware that childhood is being reshaped by forces whose mainspring is not necessarily the best interests of the child. At the same time the public is even more aware that many of the corrosive social problems affecting their quality of life have their genesis in the changing ecology of childhood.

The history of childhood

It can be helpful to have some knowledge of the history of childhood so we understand the messages from the past, which influence our way of thinking about children in the twenty-first century. There seems to be a split in the construction of childhood, an ongoing narrative between the child as 'innocent victim' and the child as a 'little devil'.

In his book *Centuries of Childhood* (1960) Aries suggested that the first recognition and interest in childhood emerged in the sixteenth and seventeenth centuries when childhood was seen as a time of innocence and sweetness. This was the coddling period. There was a reaction to 'coddling' in the seventeenth century largely led by churchmen and pedagogues. Aries defined this as the moralistic period. Children were perceived as fragile creatures who needed to be both safeguarded and reformed.

These ideas laid the groundwork for the development of child psychology and greatly influenced ideas about childhood and child rearing up to contemporary times. These two concepts of childhood, coddling and disciplining, passed into family life. Many rhymes and stories for children define these two concepts.

This is an example of a coddling rhyme:

Alie blie alie balie bee
Sittin' on your mammie's knee:
Greetin' from another bawbee
To buy sugar candy.

Hush-a-bye, baby,
The beggar shan't have 'ee
No more shall the maggoty-pie;
The rooks nor the ravens,
Shan't carry 'ee to heaven,
So hush-a-bye-baby, bye-bye.

Down with the lambs,
Up with the lark,
Run to bed children
Before it gets dark.

And here is a very 'troublesome' girl! But, alas, too late to reform:

The Giddy Girl

Miss Helen was always too giddy to heed
What her mother had told her to shun
For frequently, over the street in full speed,
She would cross where the carriages run.

And out she would go to a very deep well
To look at the water below:
How naughty! To run to a dangerous well,
Where her mother forbade her to go!

One morning intending to take but one peep,
Her foot slipped away from the ground;
Unhappy misfortune! The water was deep,
And giddy Miss Helen was drowned.

The Wee Wee Mannie describes a boy's attempt to control his cow and the strategies he uses on the advice of his mother. Perhaps it mirrors the way his mother disciplines her son – when empathy for others doesn't work the threat of death makes for a compliant cow and a compliant son.

The Wee Wee Mannie

Once upon a time when all big folk were little ones and all lies were true, there was a wee wee Mannie that had a big big Coo. And out he went one morning and said:

> Hold still my Coo my hinny
> Hold still my hinny my Coo,
> And ye shall have for your dinner,
> What but a milk white-doo.

But the big big Coo wouldn't hold still. 'Hout!' said the wee wee Mannie.

> Hold still, my Coo, my dearie
> And fill my bucket with milk
> And if ye'll no' be contrary
> I'll give ye a gown of silk.

But the big big Coo wouldn't hold still. 'Look at that now!' said the wee wee Mannie.

> What's a wee wee Mannie to do
> With such a contrary Coo?

So off he went to his mother at the house. 'Mother,' he said, 'Coo won't stand still and wee wee Mannie can't milk big big Coo.'
'Hout!' says his mother. 'Take a stick and beat the Coo.'
So off he went to get a stick from a tree and said,

> Break stick break
> And I'll gi'e ye a cake.

But the stick wouldn't break so back he went to the house.
'Mother,' he said, 'Coo won't hold still, stick won't break, wee wee Mannie can't beat big big Coo.'
'Hout!' says his mother. 'Go to the butcher and bid him kill the Coo.'

So off he went to the butcher and said,

Butcher, kill the big big Coo
She'll give me no more milk noo.

But the butcher wouldn't kill the Coo without a silver penny so back the Mannie went to the house. 'Mother,' says he, 'Coo won't hold still, stick won't break, Butcher won't kill without a silver penny, and wee wee Mannie can't milk big big Coo.'

'Well,' says his mother, 'go to the Coo and tell her there's a weary weary lady with long yellow hair weeping for a sup o' milk.'

So off he went and told the Coo but she wouldn't hold still so back he went and told his mother.

'Well,' said his mother, 'tell the big big Coo there's a sharp sharp sword at the belt of the fine fine laddie from the wars who sits beside the weary weary lady with the golden hair and she is weeping for a sup o' milk.'

And he told the big big Coo but she wouldn't hold still.

'Then,' said his mother 'run quick and tell her that her head's going to be cut off by the sharp sharp sword in the hands of the fine fine laddie if she doesn't give the sup o' milk the weary weary lady weeps for.'

And the wee wee Mannie went off and told the big big Coo.

And when the Coo saw the glint of the sharp sharp sword in the hand of the fine fine laddie come from the wars and the weary weary lady weeping for a sup o' milk she thought she'd better hold still; so wee wee Mannie milked the big big Coo and the weary weary lady with the golden hair hushed her weeping and got her cup o' milk and the fine fine laddie new come from the wars put by his sharp sharp sword and all went well that didn't go ill.

The 'care and control' of children

Marina Warner, in her book *Managing Monsters* (1994), describes childhood as 'special and magical, precious and dangerous at once' (p.35). In our society this special sphere of childhood has grown as a social concept, as a market possibility, as an area of research, as a problem.

She considers that contemporary child mythology enshrines children to meet adult desires and dreams and we call children 'little devils', 'little monsters', 'little beasts' with the full ambiguous force of the terms, all the complications of love and longing, repulsion and fear.

Perhaps these two definitions of children and adolescents experiencing problems mirror the term 'care and control' in that adults 'care' for troubled children and adolescents but seek to 'control' troublesome behaviour in that group. There is a difference in attitude between being concerned 'for' a child as opposed to being concerned 'about' a child.

The term 'troubled' is often used to describe children and adolescents who are offered help and support through Child Mental Health Services or Social Services because of their difficult life circumstances. In this case, the child is passive, a victim, who has been at the receiving end of hurt or harm.

'Troublesome' is the term often used to describe deviant behaviour that is a public concern. The child involved in 'troublesome' conduct is considered to be active and a perpetrator, and attention is focused on this aspect of self-presentation.

Children as social problems

Corsaro in *The Sociology of Childhood* (1997) describes two ways in which children are viewed as social problems: the Bogeyman Syndrome and Blaming the Victim. The Bogeyman Syndrome is the general fear of the victimization of children in contemporary industrial society. This is seen in the widespread belief in certain urban legends concerning threats to children's safety as well as in the disproportional concerns about relatively rare crimes such as child abduction. Blaming the Victim refers to the tendency to hold children personally responsible for the complex social and economic forces and problems that so dramatically affect their lives.

Corsaro considers that we view children as incomplete and immature, in need of instruction, training and discipline. For this reason children are often treated as an out-group – as separate from and inferior to adults. In this way children are not seen as adults in the making or as junior selves but as inferior and not worthy of the same respect as adults.

Children under the care of the state

In a chapter in *Constructing and Reconstructing Childhood* (1990), Hendrick reviewed the constructions and reconstructions of British childhood from 1800 to the present day. He described the emergence of the Family Child and the Public Child after the Second World War and the new emphasis given to the home environment for children who had been taken into care by the local authority. He suggested that reformers have usually treated children as 'things', as problems, but rarely as human beings with personality and integrity. 'Troubled' and 'troublesome' children can become the responsibility of the state by entering the care system.

A Social Services Inspectorate Report, *When Leaving Home is also Leaving Care* (1997), quoted the following UK statistics:

- More than 75 per cent of care leavers have no academic qualifications of any kind.

- More than 50 per cent of young people leaving care after the age of 16 are unemployed.

- Seventeen per cent of young women leaving care are pregnant or already mothers.

- Twenty-three per cent of adult prisoners and 38 per cent of young prisoners have been in care.

- Thirty per cent of young homeless people have been in care.

Sadly, there has been little change in the statistics since this report.

Barriers to reform

Joseph Rowntree-funded research published in March 2000 identified the following barriers to change in the UK context:

- public attitudes towards children generally and looked after children in particular

- the human rights of children are often not the dominant value base of social services departments

- the concept of 'being a good parent' is not one that local authorities have generally applied to their relationship with looked after children

- responses to children's needs are often dominated by a service-led approach

- social workers are often not able to fulfil the role that children want from them.

In the context of this report 'being a good parent' has not really been considered as part of a social worker's task. For example, a 'good parent' might fight to get their child in a particular school because of its reputation for academic success, but a social worker does not necessarily perceive this as a role for his or her support of a child in care who might benefit from such a schooling.

Service-led approaches mean that the child in care is offered a service generated by the policies of a social work department which might not be congruent with that particular child's personal needs. For example, a child might want to stay with foster carers with whom he or she has made a strong attachment, but the policy of the department is to place children for adoption so the child is moved on to another family.

'Looked after' children say that they want to be like other children and not considered as 'different' or stand out at school or with their peers. They expect their social worker to offer a parenting role. They want constant support but not to see so many professional people like psychologists, psychiatrists and paediatricians, which reinforces their difference from other children.

The upbringing of children

The upbringing of children can be viewed through managing these aspects of identity in which some children are viewed as 'troubled', in need of help and support, or 'troublesome', in need of punishment and control. This simplistic view of the care of children might inhibit our understanding of children as people and thus place them on the 'outside' and as a source of social problems, because they do not feel included. It is notable that children are not often asked for their opinions about how they should be treated. Perhaps we should start to think about our relationship with children through the basic concepts of the UN Convention on the Rights of the Child. There are four main principles:

- non-discrimination

- best interests of the child

- the right to life, survival and development

- the views of the child.

This would seem to be a more appropriate basis for supporting children, and perhaps if we are to really understand the perspectives of children we should start by entering their world through sharing the processes by which they make sense of their environment. Pretend play and play as narrative are the ways children make sense of their world. They play aspects of their lived environment through role-play and enactment and making imaginary stories with toys and objects to represent their understanding of the relationships between people in their world. Play is the medium of communication because it is the way children structure their experiences. So let us all learn to play with children to find out what they think and feel.

Understanding play

Huizinga (1949) suggested that in play there was something 'at play' which transcended the immediate needs of life and imparted meaning to the action. It was a stepping out of 'real life' into a temporary sphere of activity. At the same time there was an intensity and absorption in play. Play was distinct from ordinary life both as to its locality and duration. There were limits to play: it began, then it was over. Play assumed a fixed form as a cultural phenomenon. Once played it endured as a new-found creation of the mind retained by the memory. It was transmitted, it became tradition.

These play traditions can be the cultural cement in families reinforcing attachments. That peek-a-boo game, the bedtime rituals of 'Good night, sleep tight, don't let the bugs bite.' Silly games, names for each other, pretend stories about family pets all create a family culture and a safe place for children to thrive. When families are reconstituted, perhaps through adoption or stepfamilies, new rituals can be developed to support the changes so that everybody has a place and a role in the new family. Here are some silly rhymes and jokes, which can become part of a family play routine to bind children and adults together through shared laughter and fun. Question and answer play starts the communication.

Play Touching Body Parts

Brow of knowledge,
Eye of life.
Scent bottle,
Penknife.
Cheek cherry,
Neck of grace,
Chin of pluck,
That's your face.
Shoulder of mutton,
Chest of fat,
Vinegar bottle,
Mustard pot,
That's my little boy/girl.

Jokes

What's frozen water?
Ice.
What's frozen cream?
Ice cream.
What's frozen tea?
Iced tea.
What's frozen ink?
Iced ink.
Then take a bath!

What do you call an igloo without a toilet?
An ig.

Teacher: If you had 10p and you asked your dad for another 10p how much would you have?
Boy: Er, 10p, sir.
Teacher: You don't know your arithmetic, boy!
Boy: You don't know my dad, sir.

Rhyme for Two People

I'm not, says she,
So braw, says she,
Nor yet, says she,
So big, says she,
But I'll go, says she,
To Perth, says she,
And get, says she,
A man, says she,
And then, says she,
I'll be, says she,
As good, says she,
As you, says she.

Rhyme for Bedtime

Come, let's to bed
Says Sleepy-Head;
Tarry awhile, says Slow;
Put on the pot,
Says Greedy-gut,
We'll sup before we go.

And my favourite song, be it the original version written by Thomas Dekker or the Beatles version. A true coddling lullaby:

Golden slumbers kiss your eyes
Smiles awake you when you rise,
Sleep pretty darling, do not cry,
And I will sing a lullabye.

Care is heavy, therefore sleep you;
You are care, and care must keep you,
Sleep pretty darlings do not cry,
And I will sing a lullabye.

Characteristics of play

Johnson, Christie and Yawkey (1999) describe five characteristics of play that help us understand the process.

1. The play frame – This separates play from everyday experience. Within the play frame the internal reality of 'playing' takes precedence over external reality.

2. Play motivation – This is an intrinsic characteristic originating in the individual; activities are pursued for their own sake.

3. The importance of process over product – Children's attention during play focuses on the activity itself, rather than the goals of the activity. The resulting absence of pressure tends to make play more flexible than goal-oriented behaviour.

4. Free choice – For young children this is an important element of their understanding of play; this appears to become less important in older children.

5. Positive affect – Usually accompanied by signs of pleasure and enjoyment, play is a valued activity even when it appears less pleasurable. The apprehension experienced by a child during play, for example when climbing to the top of the slide, may in itself be pleasurable, as the repetition of such activities suggests.

Pretend play

There are many terms for pretend play such as symbolic, make-believe, dramatic or fantasy play. All these terms define a specific process distinguished from other forms of play (practice, sensori-motor, functional, games with rules) by the criteria of non-literal play. It is the 'as if' function of pretend play which distinguishes its quality. Children engage in pretend play when they give identities and functions to objects and people that they do not possess in reality. These identities and functions then transform and transcend reality.

Pretend play usually begins in the second half of the second year when children start to do simple actions like pretending to eat with toy spoons and pouring out pretend drinks. The precursor for this kind of play is the parent/carer–child interaction when the child is about one year old. The adult signals to the child through exaggeration, increased gazing and smiling at the child that they are not acting seriously but pretending. Children who have not yet learned to pretend themselves still show sensitivity to the adult's pretence actions; they gaze and smile more toward the adult when she pretends than when she does a proper serious action (Richert, Lillard and Vaish 2002). Children up to four years of age will often use a body part as a substitute for an object in pretend play. For example, when pretending to brush their teeth they will use the index finger to represent the toothbrush. Four-year-olds will mime the toothbrush and as children develop they can develop structured sequences in their play and storytelling.

Novosyolova (1991) developed a scheme of the forms of action occurring during the development of play. This scheme describes four forms of action. In the first year of life there is *familiarizing play* which includes exploring the toy, actions with the toy and actions with the toy as a tool. In the second and third years of life *imaginative play* and *thematic imaginative play* develop. The content of this play is drawn from the child's life experience and the play is about everyday situations. Playful actions are often repeated, so the child puts a doll to bed, covers it with a blanket, then takes it out of the bed, puts it back in the bed and so on. This play can use toys, replacement objects, 'as if' actions and actions with imaginary objects. From three to seven years *thematic role-play* emerges. There is an emotional expression of role through the use of the toy, so, for example, the child plays mother putting the doll to bed and talks to the doll, connecting speech with the role taken. There is often role-discussion with other children who are playing. Novosyolova states that children combine individual events from everyday life with imaginary situations. These may sometimes even take on a fairy-tale character, yet they are always based on children's own personal experience.

Brian, aged five, made the following story with small toys and slime.

The Damp Place

The damp place was a bad place but it has now turned good because Brian wanted it good.
In the pond is a ball that wasn't well and all the creatures in the pond wasn't well.
This was an alien and he wasn't well and a dinosaur.
The pond made them ill because it had bad poison and germs in it.
It is not scary but people get ill because it is dirty.
The pond got full with hundreds and hundreds of creatures.
And in the end they all died so the pond was empty.
The End.

He is using the toys to create an imaginary story and elements of the story define the way he represents his world at that particular time when he was playing with me. It is important to remember that children use pretend play to experiment with their ideas about the worst things and the best things in their world as well as the worst people and the best people. They do not necessarily wish to carry these stories into their lived world but perhaps find comfort in experimenting with ideas in the presence of a supportive adult who can keep them safe enough to think the unthinkable.

An example is a story by Ted, aged five, who was to move to a permanent family after some time in care. He told everyone how happy he was to move and had no fears at all. His story in play expressed his excitement but also his anxieties.

> Ted was looking for a new mum and dad.
> He was in a police car.
> Another car came along with Ted's new mum and dad.
> They saw Ted in the police car and called out to him.
> And he was so pleased to get a new mum and dad.
> Somebody took Ted away because they didn't want him to have a new mum and dad.
> They took Ted to jail.
> Ted was crying.
> The door shuts and Ted is trapped in the jail.
> The fire engine came to rescue Ted.
> The police were sorry and said, 'You go back to your new mum and dad.'
> Ted is flying in the fire engine.
> 'Hello I'm lost,' says Ted.
> 'The fire burnt down my new mum's home.'
> Ted is inside the house on the roof and he falls off.
> But doesn't get hurt.
> The fire was put out and Ted went down.
> All the cars went away.
> And that's the end of the story.

This is a pretend story but it shows a hero who is not certain about adults and whether they will care for him. Are they strong enough to combat external events and will Ted ever get to find them in the first place? At the end of the story it is not clear if the hero's new mum and dad will be able to care for him. He survives the fire, the cars go away and that is as much as Ted can imagine at this moment. This was Ted's symbolic experiment with imaginative choices in his playing world, distanced from the consequences of those choices in his reality world. So we stay with the story as it is. Ted was able to describe his anxieties in his play and stories but not in general conversation with his carers or social worker. To them he appeared to be coping well with the move to a new family so it was helpful to discuss Ted's anxieties with his present carers and new family so they were aware of his fears.

When children play imaginatively, in whatever context, they create a fictional world which can be a way of making sense of their lived life. Vandenberg (1986) states that to be human and live in a meaningful way within a culture requires that we live in and through a very sophisticated abstract system that is largely imaginary. Our social relationships and our understanding of our work and our culture depend on our understanding of these systems of communication, both verbal and non-verbal. Jokes, irony, skills of persuasion and figures of speech are all part of this system as well as non-verbal signals and signs like eye contact and smiling.

Pretend play as narrative

Telling stories as a means of constructing social meaning is embedded in all human cultures and traditions and it may well be a biological given (Bruner 1990). Once children have begun to acquire language they show an ability to organize their experience in a narrative form. It is through these narratives that children express their unique way of thinking and feeling about themselves, their own personal voice, and what it is like to be in their world. So Ted's world when he told me his story was one which contained his wishes and fears and expressed the unknown future with all his desires, longings and terrors. Play is the natural way for children to construct coherence and meaning which is the purpose of narrative. From a narrative perspective the invitation to play is no more than the posing of the autobiographical request, 'tell me your story'.

Engel (1995) says that it is also important to recognize that stories not only reconstruct experience and communicate experience but they *are* experience and through the stories we tell, especially the stories we tell about ourselves, we construct ourselves. At any given moment how we

behave, feel and experience ourselves grows in part out of the self we
have woven together from all our past experiences and imaginings about
the future.

Adult and child playing together

There is a very special quality to a relationship based on storytelling.
There is a storyteller and a listener and the story acts in the middle as a
way to negotiate a shared meaning between the two. I have stated
elsewhere (Cattanach 1997) that in play therapy children tell stories as
containers for their experiences, constructed into the fictional narrative
of a story. There is a playfulness in the communication, whatever the
horror of the story, and the roles of storyteller and listener both have an
equal function as the story emerges in the space between the two. There
has to be a spark of recognition between storyteller and listener as the
story unfolds. The equality in the relationship facilitates the unfolding of
the story. Together the adult and child share the drama of the story as the
meaning emerges. The not knowing–knowing adult does not displace
this process with a hierarchy of adult 'knowledge' but learns to listen in a
way that supports the unfolding of the tale. The story can be acknowledged by the adult who as listener values what is presented, or the child
and adult can deconstruct and then reconstruct the story to the satisfaction of the child if new options seem desirable. This is defined as a
polyvocal collaboration. The aim is not to locate a solution or a new story
but to generate a range of new options.

Mary, aged four, likes to play with a witch doll. The doll is the 'bad'
witch. At the end of the story Mary thought of many endings. So the 'bad
witch' can be dead never to come alive again, be dead but come alive, go
to prison, change into a good witch. She didn't have to make a choice just
to tell me what might happen, that there were options.

Goolishian (1990) describes the relationship between therapist and
child. He states that to maintain a position of openness and uncertainty in
a therapeutic conversation requires the skill and patience of an experienced therapist. The therapist's not knowing does not mean the dissolu-
tion or abandonment of prior knowledge but rather its questioning. Not
knowing refers to what I do with what I know. This equally applies to the
parent/carer of the child, or a professional worker forging a relationship.

The knowledge base for parent/carer, professional worker and therapist will be different but all have a value for the child if the adult can critically evaluate their knowledge base and define what can support the development of the child as they play together.

From my perspective as a play therapist my knowledge base comes from a variety of sources, theory, training, clinical and life experiences, knowledge of empirical research, intuition, empathy and shared knowledge with other colleagues. This knowledge base has to be used hermeneutically so that it enriches the client's understanding rather than closing it off by imposing an 'expert opinion'. So knowledge is brought to the therapeutic conversation as part of the desire to understand more. The knowledge base of the parent/carer or other professional workers is equally valid. It is helpful if the adult is aware and can define their skills, which would support the relationship between child and adult, and continually monitor the relationship to ensure that the needs of the child are paramount.

Play as a cultural routine

The way the adult negotiates playing with the child is crucial to the co-working of the interaction. If the structure is clear, the play becomes another cultural routine, which gives the child a sense of belonging, creating a place where the child has a role and responsibilities. Corsaro (1997) describes a cultural routine as a place where the child has the security and shared understanding of belonging to a social group. Because the routine is predictable this provides a framework within which a wide range of sociocultural knowledge can be produced, displayed and interpreted.

These routines serve as anchors, which enable the child to deal with ambiguities, the unexpected and the problematic, while remaining within the confines of everyday life. Participation in cultural routines begins early with, for example, simple participation in the game of peek-a-boo. Initially the child learns a set of predictable rules that make up the game, then they learn that embellishment of the rules is possible as the play routine develops. Initially in these routines the games often proceed on an 'as if' assumption which means that the adult assumes that the child is capable of social interaction until the child gradually learns to be socially competent and can fully participate in these social routines.

If we explore our pretend play together as a cultural routine then the structure of the play must be well described to the child. The rules and boundaries are vital to the safety of the relationship and clarify the roles and responsibility for both adult and child. The child needs to feel safe with the adult but must also feel confident that the adult can enter his play world and help make sense of the confusion and misunderstandings which might be creating difficulties for the child. In this way the adult together with the child mediate some satisfactory meaning that is congruent with the child's social world. As the routines of pretend play are learnt and experienced, the child expands the meanings of the play and stories and learns more complex social communication.

The mediating materials are the play, story-making with toys and objects and stories the therapist tells or reads which extends the child's individual experience to a cultural generality. The cultural routines are also established and reinforced through the narratives spoken between the adult and child during their time together. Children enjoy their mastery over the space, structure, and the time spent with the adult, and are very strict that all the routine is maintained. It is often while setting up the area for play that the child will tell an imaginary story or narrate a family or school situation.

The playing space

When children engage in pretend play they find a place where they feel safe enough to play. Children play in spaces on the borders of everyday life, perhaps under the table, down in the den at the bottom of the garden, in their bedroom, but in spaces where they can still keep contact with their family or social group. I still fondly remember my little attic room where I played school and especially the lock on the door so I could keep my bossy sister out.

Bateson (1972) states that before engaging in imaginative play children must establish a play 'frame' or context to let others know that what is happening is play; that it is not real. This is usually done by smiling and laughing. In pretend play children operate on two levels; at one level they are involved in their pretend roles and focus on the make-believe meaning of objects and actions. At the same time they are aware of their own identities, the other players' identities and the real-life meaning of the objects and actions used in the play.

In everyday life autistic children hardly engage in spontaneous pretend play but studies (Lewis and Boucher 1988; Libby *et al.* 1997) found that autistic children were able to use pretend play when it was scaffolded and elicited through modelling and instruction to imitate in highly supportive social contexts. I remember working in the Netherlands with a group of autistic adolescents who were able to play scenes of café life once the structure had been modelled for them. They could not spontaneously develop the narrative but enjoyed playing people in a café drinking coffee. They took great comfort each week from the repetition of the scene, which created a cultural routine for the group with each individual clear about their role in the scene.

As a play therapist, if I am meeting children in their home environment, we choose a place to play which does not interrupt the flow of activity in the home. So perhaps the child's bedroom or dining room. There is nothing worse than depriving the rest of the household of their routine activities by taking the central room in the house. Parents or carers could find a special place and time in the house for pretend play and make it part of family life for the child or children. This can support attachment between adult and child, giving the child affirmation that what they play is interesting for the adult.

If professional workers are using rooms or a playroom away from the home environment, it is important that the space is nurturing for the child. I always use a special blue mat to sit on with the child and this delineates the playing area. The mat is large enough to seat the child, myself and the toys. It is important in each environment to have a playing place and a non-playing space in the same room so the child can stop playing without leaving the room. This gives clarity about when the child is playing and when the play is over or stopped for a while.

Rules when playing together

It is important to have rules when adult and child play together. The rules are about who is responsible for what. The adult will bring the toys and will be responsible for bringing the same toys each time and keeping them safe meanwhile. Parents/carers may want to select some special toys and objects for this special time of play with the child and these can be kept separate from the general toys in the household, and in a special place. Many children want to set out the place and the space because it is perhaps one environment over which they can gain mastery. Most of the children I see want to put the mat out and organize our sitting together. Play is the child's world and one of the few places where they have control over the setting and can choose the play objects and set the scene.

The child is expected to play and make stories. That is their responsibility. The adult is expected to listen to the child and also participate in the play at the request of the child. The adult is responsible for bringing the toys and other play materials and for making sure the same toys are available for each play session. Professional workers may want to have their own set of toys because general toys kept in a play room can get lost and broken and do not hold the same value for the child as toys which are special for the playing adult.

Both child and adult are responsible for rules of behaviour. No hitting and hurting, respect for body boundaries, respect for each other. The structure is very important for the child so they know what is expected and, feeling safe, they can develop their play in the space, through time, with toys and objects.

Toys for pretend play

The choice of toys to encourage children to play together with an adult is largely determined by the preferences of the players and the environment where the play takes place. If the adult is taking toys to the child then the selection has to be limited but should include materials for sensory play, figures for story-making and art materials. If the meetings are in a playroom or at home then the choices are less limited. However, some children can be overwhelmed by too much stimulation, so too many toys can be unhelpful. A small box of interesting toys is as valuable as a playroom full of objects randomly selected. The play between child and adult is special so the same toys should always be there at each playtime. There is nothing worse for a child than to find a key toy is missing or broken, so one of the rules should be for the adult to keep the toys safe.

Suggestions for playing materials include the following:

SENSORY MATERIALS

Slime, Play Doh, clay, sand and bubbles are a stimulus for sensory play. Children often start their pretend play with sensory play. It seems to focus children into the playing mode. Sometimes the sensory materials become part of a pretend story so figures are placed in slime or sand or Play Doh and the materials are often used as a metaphor for the 'messiness' in the children's lives. John, aged four, made a pond with pink slime, placed small figures in the slime, and told the following story:

> Once upon a time there was a pond.
> It was a scary place.
> The people were scary and the pond.
> The pond was very cold.
> There was an alien in the pond
> But it was dead.
> A foot was in the pond and it was all messy.
> A lizard came there and a dinosaur
> And they all had a swim.

John had just moved to an adoptive family and perhaps his story expressed what that might be like for him trying to cope with new people, a new place and new rules.

SMALL FIGURES

A selection of small figures facilitate story-making and might include the following.

A group of family figures

If children have lived in several families there should be enough figures to represent this. The Simpson family are often used by children in family stories. Include ethnically diverse figures.

Magical figures

Include dragons and witches, knights and current figures from film and television. I note that ninja turtles are back in favour so I can retrieve them from storage.

Animals, wild and domestic

Lions, tigers, elephants, foxes, hares, penguins and so forth. Dogs, cats, other domestic animals, rabbits, farm animals and donkeys are popular.

Cars and things

Cars are very important objects denoting for many children a safe place to be; cars also move from place to place. Unattached children often make stories with cars being driven with no drivers, no people around. This is often repetitive play before the child learns to develop a story. Planes, helicopters and skateboards all denote movement.

The environment

Small objects to denote surroundings, trees, a bench, signs etc., and indoors, a bed, a chair, sofa, a potty, etc.

This is a story from Stuart, aged seven, using small figures:

The Witch Murders

There was a witch called Madge,
And she bites people.
She bit Bart Simpson's dad
And killed him and ate him up.
She buried him in sand.
Then Madge ate a man
Then a cow then a bat then a dog
Then a metal dog then a snake
Then a fish then a sheep
Then Bart Simpson then a huge snake
Then a girl then a big snake and a caterpillar.
Then a knight killed her to death
And brought all the people back alive.

DOLLS AND PUPPETS

Dolls with clothes and feeding bottles, etc. Hand puppets which are easy to manipulate. Animal puppets can include crocodiles, wolves and dogs. Include fierce creatures and warm and loving figures.

DRESSING-UP CLOTHES

These can include adult clothes as well as specific costumes like Spiderman, etc., also shoes, bags, hats and lots of interesting material to make cloaks, etc.

MATERIALS FOR DRAWING AND PAINTING
Paint, a variety of crayons and pastels, coloured paper and tactile paper masks to draw on.

The adult as storyteller

When I listen to the stories children make up in play I am often reminded of folk tales or stories which are congruent with what the child has invented. I might then tell the story to the child, because to know that other people have told stories with similar themes can help the child feel like everybody else rather than the only person in the world who has their life experiences or who can tell such stories.

I see two boys who are nine years old and they are at the stage of telling gruesome stories and trying out shock tactics. They have been in trouble for swearing at the wrong people in the wrong places. We explore these issues as they play and they make up gruesome stories to shock themselves and me. I told them the story of the boy on the ice. They were impressed and asked if the story was true. 'Who knows,' I said, 'it's a story.' We all laughed; there were others out there who had our sense of the gruesome.

Keep a Cool Head

He was a great lad for telling stories, he had a great lot of stories, and it was New Year's Day, ice came on the loch and all the young boys came down there skating.

They were all out there, ice on the loch, and they were skating and then one of the boys got a bit too far out, and in the middle of the loch the ice was soft, and it broke with him and he went down, down in a hole, and the other edge of the ice just caught him under the chin.

He slid away under the ice till he came to another hole, and his head did the same on top of the ice, and when they came together there his head just stuck on again… The frost was that strong it just froze his head on again.

In the evening then they were sitting around the hearth telling stories, and the boy was there too, and he was getting rid of some of the cold with his dip in the cold water, you know, and he starts to sneeze.

As he was going to blow his nose, they just blow their nose with their fingers then, you know, as he was going to blow his nose and with the heat, it kind of thawed the ice about his neck, you know, he aimed his head and it shot right into the fire.

Sarah, aged six, liked to end her play with a funny story and always the same story because this was a predictable moment in a turbulent life. It is a funny, silly story and made us laugh about speaking before thinking of consequences. Sarah liked to join in when each wish was gone so now we tell the story together.

The Three Wishes

A little man came to a wee house on a wet day and asked for supper.

They gave him a bowl of soup and some bread and when he went they gave him a little round thing and said it would give him three wishes.

So the next morning the man said, 'Soup again, I wish I had a pudding for a change.'

And there was a pudding.

'Oh you fool,' said his wife. 'One wish gone, I wish the pudding was on your head!'

And it was.

'That's two wishes gone,' said the man.

The wife said, 'You ought to have wished for a gold bar or anything.'

'I wish the pudding was off my head,' said the man.

And that was the three wishes gone.

The importance of pretend play and cognitive competence

There is a concept of children's play which defines it as trivial, unimportant and that the child should grow up and leave such nonsense behind. However, as research into pretend play evolves, it is clear that pretend play is key to the cognitive competence of the child.

Bergen (2002) refers to the growing body of evidence supporting the many connections between cognitive competence and high-quality pretend play. If children lack opportunities to experience such play, their long-term capacities related to metacognition, problem solving and social cognition, as well as to academic areas such as literacy, mathematics and science, may be diminished. These complex and multidimensional skills involving many areas of the brain are most likely to thrive in an atmosphere rich in high-quality pretend play.

CHAPTER 2

How Did I Begin?

Making sense of the universe

Where did I come from? A philosophical question we all ask. Every culture has stories of their origins, making sense of the vastness of the universe and their place within it.

Frayn (2006) states that when we look up into the clear night sky we are looking into chaos, a vague cloud of solidified droplets, arranged in patterns that have no discernible regularity, but the relationship within this cloud, however irregular, however incomprehensible, seems to remain unchanged night after night, year after year, century after century, millennium after millennium, and gradually our skill at metaphor and our ability to see shape where no shape is offered enables us to map even this final wilderness. We slowly learn to read into it similarities to the regular objects of the terrestrial world.

We all tell stories about the universe, the meaning of the stars, black holes, the clouds, and try to connect them to our lives and personal histories. When we play with children who are struggling to find a place for themselves we can start with play and stories about the world 'out there' as a way to begin our personal history. I often ask children to imagine, perhaps draw a picture, of where they came from before they were born. It's a pretend story. Did they fly in through the air, or crawl out of the sea or perhaps burst in from a comet? It can be great fun to imagine, perhaps, Superboy/Supergirl flying through the air. A sort of being before becoming. Chloe, aged seven, described herself as a baby ghost before she was born. When I think of my play and conversations with Chloe it reminds me of the following conversation of two Dogrib Indians (from Canada) looking at a constellation. It defines a relationship between two friends sharing their thoughts about the constellations through the playful give and take of a conversation.

A Dogrib Conversation While Pointing at a Constellation

'Somebody's chasing it.'

'Hey – no.'

'It's true.'

'Which?'

'That one there. I'm pointing at it. Get behind me. Look past my hand.'

'Let me see.'

'See it?'

'Yes, who's chasing it?'

'Somebody always is. It's called The-One-Always-Chased.'

'Who's chasing it now?'

'Some other one.'

'Who?'

'The One-Who-Chases.'

'One time I was out walking. Out at night. I heard a loud flint scrape.'

'Flint scrape?'

'Yes and I looked up to the sky.'

'The sound travelled down to you?'

'Yes, a flint scrape.'

'It was him. The One-Who-Chases. It wasn't the other one.'

'The other one wouldn't stop to make a fire like that. He'd be found out.'

Together they are humanizing the constellations with ideas from their own cultural understanding of their world. For hunters the one who chases and the one always chased are strong connecting images, as is the making of fire with flint sparks. Together they are making a story which identifies them in the vastness of the universe and defines objects in the universe as a way of sharing their understanding of what it is to be alive. It is this imaginative give and take in conversation which is a model for the way adult and child might play together, sharing thoughts and ideas about their place in the world. We might use toys and objects, sand and water to define our imaginary worlds and this is a way to begin our narratives of the self. J, aged seven, narrated his universe:

The space ship has come from the dark.
It will go down the land.
Nobody is inside it.
It lands on the water very quietly.
The crocodile is walking in the water.

The space ship flew in the air.
Then it came down in the water.
The water splashed the space ship.
The water went all over the space ship.
The crocodile is in the sea.
The crocodile is nice.
He is kind.
He doesn't bite people.
He has no mum and dad.
He has no children.
He lives on his own.
It is sad.

J's was a desolate universe. Ships emerged from space, all unoccupied, and the earth was dangerous and isolated. The nice crocodile was isolated and alone in a dangerous world.

Broks (2003) states that from a neuroscience perspective we are all divided and discontinuous. The mental processes underlying our sense of self – feelings, thoughts, memories – are scattered through different zones of the brain. There is no special point of convergence. No cockpit of the soul. No soul-pilot. They come together as a work of fiction. A human being is a storytelling machine. The self is a story.

Creation stories

All cultures have creation stories and they offer an interesting perspective on how different cultures express the beginning of the world through metaphor and striking images. There are times when children like to hear such stories from their own and other cultures as they play making their own worlds.

The Salishan-Sahaptin tribe from North America use the striking image of a tree as the connection between the three worlds of sky, earth and underworld. This is a soothing story to tell for children who feel dislocated by their experiences.

Making the World and People

The chief above made the earth. It was small at first, and he let it increase in size. He continued to enlarge it and rolled it out until it was very large. Then he covered it with a white dust, which became the soil.

He made three worlds one above the other – the sky world, the earth we live on, and the underworld. All are connected by a pole or tree which passes through the middle of each.

And then he created the animals.

At last he made a man, who, however, was also a wolf. From this man's tail he made a woman. These were the first people. They were the ancestors of all the people.

This Bini story from Nigeria gives a human explanation as to why the sky is far away. This is appealing for all of us tempted by greed for food.

Why the Sky is Far Away

In the beginning the sky was very close to the earth.

In those days men did not have to till the ground because whenever they felt hungry they simply cut off a piece of the sky and ate it. But the sky grew angry because they often cut off more than they could eat and threw the leftovers onto the rubbish heap.

The sky did not want to be thrown on the rubbish heap and so he warned men that if they were not more careful in future he would move far away.

For a while everyone paid attention to the warning. But one day a greedy woman cut off an enormous piece of the sky. She ate as much as she could but was unable to finish it.

Frightened, she called her husband. But he too could not finish it. In the end they had to throw the remainder in the rubbish heap.

Then the sky became very angry indeed and rose up high far beyond the reach of men. And from then on men had to work for their living.

I often use this story about the Ainu people of Japan because it describes the hard work required to make a satisfactory world. We have to clear away all the slush to make a solid foundation to build or rebuild a safe place for ourselves in the world.

In the Beginning

In the beginning the world was slush. For the waters and the mud were all stirred in together.

All was silence, there was no sound. It was cold. There were no birds in the air. There was no living thing.

At last the Creator made a little wagtail and sent him down from his far place in the sky.

Produce the earth, he said.

The bird flew down over the black waters and the dismal swamp. He did not know what to do. He did not know how to begin.

He fluttered the water with his wings, splashed it here and there. He ran up and down in the slush with his feet and tried to trample it onto firmness. He beat on it with his tail, beating it down.

After a long time of this treading and tail-wagging a few dry places began to spear in the big ocean which now surrounds them – the island of the Ainu.

The Ainu word for earth is *mishiri*, floating land, and the wagtail is revered.

End of the world stories

There are many end of the world stories, as well as creation stories, and these myths often mirror some of the desolation expressed by children who feel unsafe.

The following White River Sioux story defines that sense of vulnerability we all experience, especially in these times of global warming and other fears of the human capacity to annihilate ourselves and the world. We all, at times, experience this vulnerability.

The End of the World

Somewhere where the prairie and the badlands meet there is a hidden cave. So hidden that no one has ever found it.

In the cave lives a woman so old that her face is like a shrivelled walnut. The old woman wears rawhide the way the Sioux dressed before the white man came. She has been sitting in the cave for more than a thousand years working on a blanket strip for her buffalo robe. She is making the strip out of porcupine quills.

Resting beside her, licking his paws, watching her all the time, is Shunka Sapa, a huge black dog. His eyes never wander from the old woman, whose teeth are worn down flat into little stumps because she has used them to flatten so many porcupine quills.

A few steps from where the old woman sits working on her blanket strip a huge fire is kept going. She lit this fire a thousand or more years ago and has kept it alive ever since. Over the fire hangs a big earthen pot. Inside the pot berry soup is boiling good and sweet and red. The soup has been boiling on the pot since the fire was lit.

Every now and then the old woman gets up and stirs the pot. She is so old and feeble it takes her a while to get up and hobble over to the fire. The moment her back is turned the huge black dog starts pulling the porcupine quills out of her blanket strip. This way she never makes any progress and her quill work remains forever unfinished.

The Sioux people used to say that if the old woman ever finishes her blanket strip then at the very moment she threads the last porcupine quill to complete this design the world will come to an end. The following African story explores man's mortality:

The Chameleon and the Lizard

When Death first entered the world men sent the chameleon to find out the cause. God told the chameleon to let men know if they threw baked porridge over a corpse it would come back to life. But the chameleon was slow to return to men and Death was rampant in their midst.

So men sent a second messenger, the lizard. The lizard reached the abode of God soon after the chameleon.

God, angered by the second message, told the lizard that men should dig a hole in the ground and bury their dead in it. On the way back the lizard overtook the chameleon and delivered his message first, and when the chameleon arrived the dead were already buried.

Thus, owing to the impatience of man, he cannot be born again.

It is interesting how similar some children's stories are to those cultural myths which define human frailty. Here are three stories from a four-year-old, a seven-year-old and a thirteen-year-old.

Ruth, aged four, describes a dangerous world:

> Bart and his sister were playing on the skateboard and two snakes came and bit them.
> They were both dead.
> The mum and dad didn't know they were dead.
> The dogs were put in a cage because they ate all the people's dinner.

Jake, aged seven, describes a terrible monster that could destroy the whole world:

The Goblin Chopper

The Goblin Chopper is a monster and he lives in bloodslime.
A crocodile goes into the blood slime and he gets trapped.
He needs blood to go on living.
The crocodile looks for a place to hide.
The Goblin Chopper hears him coming.
He is ready to chop the crocodile.
The crocodile sees his big massive teeth and thinks it is just a cave.
He goes into Goblin Chopper's mouth.
The Goblin Chopper shuts his mouth and eats the crocodile.
The Goblin Chopper opens his mouth and a lizard comes in and frogs and more lizards.
The Goblin Chopper shuts his mouth and eats the lizards and frogs.
Inside his mouth are blood, teeth, guts and stuff.
Goblin Chopper eats everything.
The Simpson family, the dinosaur family,
The Goblin Chopper catches people and things.
He keeps them in tanks until they are mouldy and then he eats them.
Families, dinosaurs, a horse, buses, vehicles, soldiers.
Everybody in the whole world.
The End.

John, aged 13, experiences the world as evil:

The Blood Lake

The aliens come out of the ground into the lake.
They are all horrible.
The pig gets eaten by the snake.
Then a dinosaur comes and rescues the pig,
Which is alive.
But the dinosaur is bad and get eaten by the alien.
So the pig is dead inside the dinosaur inside the alien.
A frog came and he just sleeps.
Then a lizard came and eats him.
The lizard gets eaten by the crocodile.
They are young, they have parents,
But the parents are at home eating maggots
And smoking fags.
They are sitting down having tea.
At night they wonder where the children are,
So they get an alien to go out in the dark.
He finds the children dead.
He gets sucked into the lake and dies.
He is dead with all the creatures.
There are lots of funerals
For all the dead people.

Starting again

When children see the world as fearful and dangerous we need to begin at the beginning and offer soothing experiences and a reliable relationship for the child to feel safe and nurtured. This can be developed using pretend play to make a nurturing relationship where the child is heard and can explore and expand their experience of the world.

If the adult is to join the child in play it is important to know how pretend play develops in childhood so we can offer play which is developmentally appropriate.

Stagnitti and Jellie (1998, p.6) have developed an excellent breakdown of the way in which children play imaginatively at various ages and stages. This can help adults playing with children to pitch their responses at an appropriate level of understanding for the child.

The development of pretend play and narrative

- *18 months – Pretend play development:* Play themes centre on body functions (e.g. drinking and sleeping). Play is short because children only pretend using one action. Children imitate what they have seen (e.g. they give teddy a drink because their mother does the same for them).

- *20 months – Pretend play development:* Play themes include events in the home (e.g. cooking). Children can now use an object as something else (e.g. a box for a car) as long as that object is physically similar. Play actions are repetitive and short; play action sequences are illogical (e.g. put the doll to bed and then wash the doll). The doll is starting to be separate from the child because the child can sit a doll with a cup for a drink.

- *24 months – Pretend play development:* Play themes include events in and out of the home (e.g. shopping, going on the bus). Play action sequences are now simple, sequential and logical. A child can use one object for several uses.

- *24 months – Narrative development:* Narrative is created by joining events to form the seed of a story. Two-year-olds use sequences of events from real life. They are not good at identifying fictional story characters, time or setting so they tell a story about themselves. There is no clear storyline, sequencing is not fully developed. Stories do not involve cause and effect. Stories lack a beginning, middle and end format. Children can sequence in a forward direction.

- *30 months – Pretend play development:* Less frequently experienced life events are included in play (e.g. visiting the zoo). Objects can be used for a lot of different functions. Play actions are detailed and logical but there is no planned storyline. Children play beside others, the doll can now wake up and the child can use an abstract doll such as a dolly peg.

- *30 months – Narrative development*: Children attempt fictional storytelling. Stories consist mainly of actions – stories are about what the characters did. They may not identify all characters in a story. While storytelling is basic, there is dominance in use of movement and intonation and volume of voice.

- *3 years – Pretend play development*: Play themes now extend beyond the child's personal experience to include events they have seen on television or in books. Children use multiple play actions and thus play for longer. Role-play is quick and children can now play with more objects, such as all the items in a doll's house.

- *3 years – Narrative development*: Children begin to develop narrative ability. Nearly half of all children at this age demonstrate the ability to use a sequence of events in a related logical way within familiar activities. Logical time sequences begin to appear in storytelling and stories begin to have a central theme.

- *3.5 years – Pretend play development*: The child starts to develop a play strategy – the child thinks what they will play before they start to play. The stimulus for playing is from the idea, not necessarily from the toys or objects they see. They can use imaginary objects and events in play and play is associated with other children.

- *3–5 years – Narrative development*: Children move from description of objects and events to temporal sequencing of actions that solve a problem. Children use goal-directed actions. Storytelling can be enhanced.

- *4 years – Pretend play development*: Children use sub-plots in their play – two stories occur in the play theme and this involves a problem (e.g. the restaurant is out of food). Children can use an object with a distinct function (e.g. a shoe) as something else (the shoe can be a car). Children begin to play co-operatively and negotiate in play and they can play several roles during the one play session.

- *5 years – Pretend play development:* Children can play any theme. They play events they have seen or never experienced. They use language to describe and embellish objects and play actions are pre-planned, organized and complex. The doll has its own character and life and, during play, the child carries out the same role.

- *5 years – Narrative development:* Most children can link events to form in a story theme and sequence events in a related logical way using fictional characters. Causality is included.

- *6 years – Pretend play development:* Play extends using language to describe events, objects, situation and characters.

- *6 years – Narrative development:* Most children possess the basic repertoire of narrative abilities.

- *8–9 years – Pretend play development:* Play extends using language to describe events, objects, situations and characters.

- *8–9 years – Narrative development:* Children tell complete stories.

- *11–12 years – Pretend play development:* Pretend play is no longer the dominant form of play. Dolls and teddies stop 'talking' to children and are often packed away, only to come out when younger children visit a household.

- *11–12 years – Narrative development:* Children reach a peak in their ability to tell oral narratives. The average child has mastered story grammar. The child has extended beyond storytelling in narrative.

Beginning to play: Retelling and playing the self

When we start a relationship with a child through playing together we can soon establish if play stages have been missed in the developmental process. Many children who have been neglected and understimulated will be struggling to use pretend play at all and all children who have reason to mistrust adults might struggle to establish a playful relationship with an adult. I start play with simple sensory experiences and often begin with a Treasure Basket, an idea adapted from Elinor Goldschmied (unpublished). This creates a basic experience for the child of playing in the presence of someone, and no talking is required to enjoy the experience. The basket can be used once a baby can sit up but can be enjoyed at any age.

Treasure Basket

Goldschmied suggested that the basket to hold the treasures should be about 36cm across and 10–12.5cm high, with a flat bottom and no handle. The basket needs to be solid so it can be leaned on without spilling. It should be filled with a collection of objects to appeal to the senses.

During the exploration of objects in the basket, the adult is always present, attentive and available, warm but not too close to crowd the child. The adult does not initiate interest in the objects but is a firm point of reference for the child. If the basket is kept at home, older children can help to collect treasures on walks or when shopping. It is important to keep the items clean and looking fresh, with changes of objects to maintain the interest of the child.

Objects should stimulate:

- touch – texture, shape, weight
- smell – variety of scents
- taste – sweet, sour
- sound – ringing, tinkling, banging, scrunching
- sight – colour, form, length, shininess.

OBJECTS FOR THE BASKET

Goldschmied did not include plastic objects because she considered them one dimensional and crude in form although nowadays some plastic objects are better produced.

- *Natural objects*: fir cones, pebbles, shells, feathers, pumice stone, corks, sponges, lemon, apple.
- *Natural materials*: wooden ball, little baskets, raffia mat, toothbrush, nailbrush, house painting brush, bone shoe horn, wooden comb.

- *Wooden objects:* small boxes, velvet-lined small boxes, small drum, rattles, bamboo whistle, coloured beads on string, wooden curtain rings, eggcup, small wooden bowl, clothes pegs.

- *Metal objects:* spoons, bunch of keys, small tins, toy trumpet, key rings, small funnel, tin lids, a triangle.

- *Leather, textiles, rubber objects:* rubber ball, length of rubber tubing, cloth bags containing herbs like lavender, leather purse, velvet cloth, leather spectacle case, bunch of coloured ribbons, tennis ball, golf ball.

- *Paper, cardboard objects:* greaseproof paper, little notebook, paper chains, small cardboard boxes, insides of lavatory rolls.

The Treasure Basket can become a family ritual or a play ritual for a professional worker and child. It can be a very soothing form of play as the objects are explored by the child with no expectation other than to handle them. The adult watches, responds and keeps the child safe from physical harm. Objects can be carefully selected so they appeal to a particular child; for instance, some metal objects would not be available for the boisterous child who might harm him or herself. Children with a literal view of the world might choose objects together with an adult and perhaps gain more pleasure in placing the objects in the basket in a pleasing spatial configuration, rather than exploring the sensory nature of the contents.

From the Treasure Basket the child and adult could begin to relate to each other through those give-and-take plays of baby and carer, starting with peek-a-boo.

Peek-a-Boo

Put a cloth over the child's head. As you pull it off say 'peek-a-boo'.

Switch roles. Or, put your hand in front of your eyes. Remove hands and call 'peek-a-boo'.

Switch roles. Or put a cloth over a toy, get the child to take off the cloth and say 'peek-a-boo'.

Peek-a-boo and other hiding and finding games teach children about rules. In peek-a-boo the basic rules are: initial contact, disappearance, reappearance and re-established contact. From these basic rules the players can make variations by vocalizing and changing the contact responses. When the child puts a cloth over a toy then removes the cloth he or she is learning about object permanence. This game also explores the boundaries between the 'real' and 'make-believe' because the hider is still present although unseen. Children begin to understand who is 'me' and who is 'not me'. You can remember the other person with your eyes closed and a person can still be present when out of sight. Understanding that 'the other' is 'not me' is critical to our understanding of our own identity.

Developmental movement

Sherbourne (1990) explores the use of developmental movement, which she describes as a nurturing experience for some children. The process mimics the normal movement development of the baby with rolling play, rocking and sliding play and finally swinging play. The adult can get the child to push them as they roll on the floor then change around, with the child rolling. The whole body movement of a roll can be a harmonious sensation for the child as one part of the body follows after another. The hip, then the shoulder or knee and the rest of the body follows. Gentle rocking and sliding can follow, perhaps ending with a gentle swing. Sherbourne calls this relationship play. The adult and child can move towards shared physical activities like pretend rowing the boat and pretend see-saws as they grasp wrists and rock backwards and forwards. It must be remembered that many children who mistrust adults would find this shared physical activity very scary, so it should not be attempted if there is any resistance from the child.

Learning about the physical self through play and rhymes

Play through the use of rhymes and games was discussed in Chapter 1. The following rhymes are specific, to help a child define themselves and their present circumstances. The first rhyme perhaps describes how a child might feel in a new home.

As I walked by myself
And talked to myself
Myself said unto me
Look to thyself
Take care of thyself
For nobody cares for thee.

I answered myself
And said to myself
In the self-same repartee
Look to thyself,
Or not to thyself
The self-same thing will be.

That acknowledged, the family might like all those nurture rhymes, which also define the physical self. I like:

Warm hand, warm,
The men have gone to plough
If you want to warm your hands,
Warm your hands now.

Brush hair, brush,
The men have gone to plough
If you want to brush your hair,
Brush your hair now.

Wash hands, wash,
The men have gone to plough
If you want to wash your hands,
Wash your hands now.
With flowers on my shoulders,
And slippers on my feet,
I'm my mother's darling;
Don't you think I'm sweet?

It is easier to encourage a child to begin to care for themselves through a fun rhyme rather than nagging. Then carers can define their task!!

The old woman must stand at the tub tub tub
The dirty clothes to rub rub rub
But when they are clean and fit to be seen
She'll dress like a lady and dance on the green.

How about dancing together?

> Dance little baby dance up high
> Never mind baby mother is nigh
> Crow and caper, caper and crow
> There little baby there you go
> Up to the ceiling down to the ground
> Backward and forward, round and round
> Dance little baby and mother shall sing
> With the merry merry rattle, ding, dong-a-ding, ding.

Finger rhymes and play can be fun too. Make up the finger play together.

> Here is a beehive,
> Where are the bees?
> Hidden away where nobody sees.
> Soon they come creeping out of the hive
> One-two-three-four-five.

> Five little mice on the pantry floor
> Seeking for breadcrumbs or something more
> Five little mice on the shelf up high
> Feasting so daintily in a pie
> But the big round eyes of the wise old cat
> See what the five little mice are at.

> Quickly she jumps but the mice run away
> And hide in their snug little holes all day
> Feasting in pantries may be very nice,
> But home is the best say the five little mice.

Skipping rhymes are skilful and with actions make great play. How to make the actions can be inventive; how do you wriggle like a jelly? This can become a family mime.

> Jelly on the plate
> Jelly on the plate
> Wiggle-waggle, wiggle-waggle
> Jelly on the plate

> Sausage in the pan
> Sausage in the pan
> Turn it round, turn it round
> Sausage in the pan

Paper on the floor
Paper on the floor
Pick it up, pick it up
Paper on the floor

Baby in the pram
Baby in the pram
Pull her out, pull her out
Baby in the pram

Burglars in the house
Burglars in the house
Kick 'em out, kick 'em out
Burglars in the house.

Then there are all those little rhymes and sayings which become part of family history. In Scotland we have a Snow-Rhyme for the winter snow:

The folk in the east
Are plucking their geese,
And sending their feathers
To our town.

And don't forget football:

My old man's a scaffie [scavenger]
He wears a scaffie's hat
He took me round the corner
To see a football match.

The ball was in the centre
Then the whistle blew
Skinny passed to Fatty
And down the wing he flew.

Fatty passed to Skinny
Skinny passed it back
Fatty took a dirty shot
And knocked the goalie flat.

Where was the goalie
When the ball was in the net?
Hanging to the floodlights
Wi' his trousers round his neck.

And a happy toast to the family which everyone can learn and shout aloud:

> Here's to you and yours
> And here's to me and mine
> And if ever me and mine
> Meets in wi' you and yours
> Me and mine'll be as good
> To you and yours
> As you and yours
> Has been to me and mine.

Older children and adolescents who missed out on a playful relationship with an adult often want to go back and experience playing, provided they trust the adult who can offer such a relationship. These young people also enjoy more outrageous humour, so perhaps create a family from the monsters in Ricky Gervais's *Flanimals* (2004). I have often used these books with their extraordinary creatures with groups of siblings to define each other and their relationships. We always end with shrieks of laughter and some role-playing, as each becomes their creature.

David Shrigley can connect adult to adolescent. This drawing from *Who I Am and What I Want* (2003) is typical.

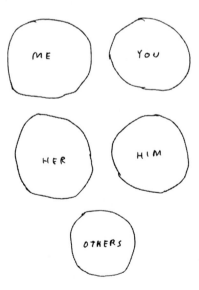

'Venn Diagram' reproduced with permission from David Shrigley (2003) Who I Am and What I Want. *London: Redstone Press.*

This kind of humour can be a starting point to play with the idea of identity, relationships in the family and with acquaintances, without offending the sensibilities of the maturing young person.

These rhymes and play are special rituals to show how a family can share affection and love and remind each other of the ties that bind. They can stay with us and be the way we remember the warm times with loved ones. So I remember:

> Night, night, sleep tight
> Don't let the bugs bite.

My father repeated this to me before bedtime and, though he is long dead, I see his smiling face as I write.

From the world story to the family story

Frayn (2006) says that we use the world to model the world. We have to. There is no other material available to us. And this is the point of our modelling – to link one piece of the world with another. This is how we survive. We look at the red blobs on the bush in front of us and we see the berries that eased our hunger yesterday. We look at that uncertain outline in the darkness and read into it the wolf that sprang at us the day before.

It is by moving from play and stories of the world to rhymes and play about ourselves and our culture that we can explore our own particular story. The Osage myth *The Children of the Sun* brings the world and the family together to make their explanation of the world.

The Children of the Sun

Way beyond the earth, a part of the Osage lived in the sky.
They wanted to know where they came from so they went to the sun.
He told them that they were his children.
Then they wandered still further and came to the moon.
She told them that she gave birth to them and that the sun was their father.
She said that they must leave the sky and go to live on earth.
They obeyed, but found the earth covered with water.
They could not return to their home in the sky
So they wept and called out but no answer came from anywhere.
They floated about in the air seeking in every direction for help
But they found none.

The animals were with them
And of these the elk inspired all creatures with confidence
Because he was the finest and most beautiful of creatures.
The Osage appealed to the elk for help.
And he dropped into the water and began to sink.
Then he called to the winds and they came from all quarters and
blew until the waters went upwards in mist.
At first only rocks were exposed and the people travelled on the
rocky places that produced no plants to eat.
Then the waters began to go down until the soft earth was
exposed.
When that happened the elk in his joy rolled over and over and all
his loose hairs clung to the soil.
The hairs grew and from them grew beans, corn potatoes and wild
turnips.
And then all the grasses and trees.

The family story

Children often describe their family story as part of a pretend play story.
Brenda, aged four, told the following story using small figures. It was her
understanding of her circumstances at that time. From creating the story,
she was able to talk with her daddy about the time she lived with her
mum. Her father gently clarified details in answer to her questions so she
understood her circumstances in an age-appropriate way.

Once upon a time there was a daddy,
He was a good daddy.
He ate all the food.
He had three children.
One boy went away
And a boy and a girl lived with him.
It was OK living with the daddy.
Before they lived with daddy,
They lived with other grown-ups.
When they lived there they were afraid.
They couldn't make dinner
So there was nothing much to eat.
They starved.
They did sex things
So they went to live with daddy.

John is seven. He was playing with family dolls and slime. He began with the pretend family story, then named figures after his parents and pushed the figures of them into slime.

> This family has two babies
> And two girls.
> They have to go in the boot of the car
> Because there is no room.
> They are going to Africa in the car.
> But they all fall out of the car
> Into the toy bag.
> The End

Then he named his parents:

> Daddy Smith is stuck in the slime
> Because he is naughty.
> And Mummy Mary.
> Ann has slime because of Daddy Smith.
> Mummy Mary couldn't stop Daddy Smith.
> He was hurting us.

He needed to include me because he felt I was contaminated by his story and his parents. From these stories his adoptive parents were able to explain more of his family history and the physical abuse he had experienced.

Sally was five and had learning difficulties. She began this session by talking about her uncles, then made a pretend story about a snake, which perhaps reflected the kind of abuse she experienced from her uncles. Then she ended by telling me what Uncle John actually did to her. The following was talk as she played with Play Doh.

> When I lived with my mum
> My uncles hurt me.
> It was a bit scary.
> Especially Uncle Rob and Uncle John.
> That's why I couldn't live with my mum.

Then she made up the following story playing with slime and toy snakes:

> There was once a snake who ate slimy stuff.
> Then he felt really sick.

Then he was sick.
And he spat the slime out of his mouth.
Then he went back home to his toy sack.

Then she stopped playing and told me about her uncles who also had some learning difficulties.

John used to take the baby's clothes off
And touch baby poo.

Sally always used pretend play to express her emotional responses to being abused and narrative to describe her uncles' behaviour. It was the pattern of our time together.

Jake was six years old. He used small dolls to tell his family story. He ends with his fear for the future. He doesn't want a new mum and dad; he wants to stay with his foster carer.

There was once a mum
And she was a naughty mum.
She was called Asha.
She swung her head around.
She took drugs with injections in her legs.
She done it on her tummy.
She shouted.
Her children thought she was very bad.
When she took drugs.
She is in the bin in jail.
There is nothing nice about my mum.
She is bad.
The children don't want a new mum and dad.

When children begin to sort out their past through play and talk they can then make a linear story melding the old and the new to find a more hopeful future. Amy is 12. She has at last found parents who want to adopt her. She has been with her birth family, three foster families and now is to be adopted. This is her story:

The Person with Very Little Brain

This person could be anyone.
She was born with very little brain and needed to get sorted.

Somebody was making fun of her saying, 'You don't have a very good brain.'
That person said that she needed somebody to cheer her up.
She was dismal because of the bad brain.
Everybody thought she was bad.
But her new family were kind.
They said she was somebody with something.
When she got older she got married, had children and a job.
When she was younger she got treatment and her brain improved.
She became kind and thoughtful for other people.
Nobody made fun of her.

My favourite hope for the future is from Suzy, aged five, and living with her mother, who struggles with mental health problems but places Suzy at the centre of her life and nurtures her well. Suzy says: 'When I stop growing it's the end of counting and I will be 20.'

We imagine the world and how it began. Our culture determines the kind of stories we can make about our beginnings. The following Hopi American Indian story soothes me when all seems hopeless.

The First World

The first world was endless space.
But first they say there was only the Creator Tokpela.
Everything else was endless space.
There was no beginning and no end,
No time, no shape, no life.
Just an immeasurable void
That had its beginning and end,
Time, shape and life in the mind of the Creator.
Then the Creator, the infinite, created the finite.
First he created his nephew Sotuknang
To carry out his plan for life in endless space.
Sotuknang did as he was ordered.
From endless space he gathered all the solid substance
And moulded it into forms
And arranged them into nine kingdoms.
One kingdom for the Creator, one for himself
And seven universes for the life to come.

'That is very good,' said the Creator.
'Now I want you to do the same with the waters.
Put them on the surfaces of these universes
So they will be divided equally among all and each.'
So Sotuknang gathered all the waters from endless space
And placed them on the universes
So each would be half solid and half water.
Sotuknang asked the Creator if his work was good.
'It is very good,' said the Creator.
'Now I want you to put the forces of air
Into peaceful movement about all.'
So Sotuknang did.
He gathered the air from endless space,
Made them into great forces
And arranged them in gentle ordered movement
Around each universe.
The Creator was pleased.
'You have done great work according to my plan.
You have created the universes,
Made them solid,
Given them water and winds
And put them in their proper places.
Now you must create Life.'
Then Sotuknang formed Spider Woman,
Who with a mixture of earth, saliva
And creative wisdom made twin gods,
To harden the earth, to animate it
With vibration and sound
And to guard it at the two poles.
After forming plants, birds and animals
In the same manner,
She made the four colours of people in three stages,
And the dawn broke
And the sun rose to greet its creatures.
Then Sotuknang made the people independently creative
By giving them speech, reproductive power
And the wisdom to use them well.

CHAPTER 3

Managing Past Traumas in the Present

Many children struggle with traumas from their past which come to haunt their present circumstances and this can impact on the quality of life at home and school. Some children have experienced abuse and hurt in their birth families; other children experience traumatic events in the course of their daily lives. A car crash, losing a beloved parent through illness or a sudden accident can all lead to a debilitating fear.

When a tragedy envelops a family they try to make sense of it all. As time passes the story shifts and moves in detail until some stories merge into the culture of the time and become folk tales or folk memories to be shared with the community. An example of such a story is the Scottish folk tale of the deaths of the seven sons of each of the three Morrison families. As endless time passed, facts shifted and changed then merged with magic to form some sort of consolation. An intolerable loss has threads of hope, so the loss becomes transformed into a story, a myth belonging to a family and a culture.

The Seven Sons of Morrison:
In Cold Winters When the Ice Was Thick

It was a very long, cold, hard winter and all the lochs were frozen. It seemed that all the folk of Dalbeattie were skating on the ice or taking part in curling matches sliding their curling stones along the ice.

There were three families of Morrison, each with seven sons all competing in the curling. They laughed and skated and whacked their curling stones all day long.

The daylight faded and all the Morrisons with their friends left the ice and began to walk back to their farms through the deep snow.

But as they walked they heard the cries of curlers on the ice and looking back towards the loch they saw crowds of fairy revellers playing on the ice. They were laughing and shouting as they slid their curling stones across the ice.

The Morrisons returned to the shore and watched. The fairies were having a wonderful time, playing and drinking, singing and sliding on the ice. They were all dressed in luminous green clothes. The fairy women began to dance as the men played their curling matches. All the three times seven sons of Morrison wanted to join in but were too frightened, until one of them couldn't contain himself and sped off across the ice to join the fairy folk. All three sets of brothers joined the fairies on the ice but their friends were too afraid or perhaps too prudent to join the fairy throng. They watched enviously from the shore.

Then suddenly above the noise and the laughter came the sound of a great crack and from end to end of the loch the ice split open. In an instant the fairies had vanished and all 21 Morrison men plunged into the deep black waters of the loch. They were drowned in an instant in front of their friends watching from the shore.

And for many centuries travellers passing the loch near the midnight hour have seen the fairy dancers dressed in green and among them the three times seven sons of Morrison on steeds of milk-white foam. They gallop among their fairy folk with spears of sedge and swords of rush. Before the morning they are gone. No blade of grass crushed, no drop of dew disturbed as they gallop away.

The Morrisons' tragedy was made into a fiction in their community. The pain of losing 21 young men from the same family as they drowned when the ice split on the loch was too much to bear. And so it became embedded in a fictional story of young men lured to their death by the fairy folk. Perhaps this brought comfort to those who are left to experience the grief of so many young men drowned. The sons of Morrison became immortal, and we picture their youth and vitality as we imagine them forever riding the waves of the loch with the fairy folk. The fantasy image merges with the reality of loss. Their tragic story is told around the fire of a winter evening as a warning to others about the dangers of ice on the loch and an expression of grief and longing when a whole generation of young men were lost to their community.

Understanding traumatic stress

Some events and experiences in our lives are so stressful that they are likely to overwhelm our capacity to cope. We seem paralysed by the events, unable to fight the experiences or leave them behind. We lose our capacity for fight or flight but somehow oscillate between the two or stay frozen.

Eisen and Goodman (1998) distinguish traumatic from stressful events in the following way: trauma seriously threatens the health or survival of the individual, it renders the individual powerless in the face of overwhelming fear or arousal, it overwhelms the individual's coping capacity and it violates basic assumptions about the environment's human and/or physical benevolence and safety.

Traumatic stress can occur whether directly experienced or witnessed. For example, a child witnessing a father's extreme violence towards her mother can be as traumatized as if she was physically attacked herself. Jamie, aged seven, told me about life with two alcoholic, violent parents. When they came home drunk they began to fight. He was terrified and flattened himself against the wall of the sitting room, pretending he was wallpaper so he wouldn't be noticed and attacked. He lived in a state of constant terror, never knowing when the next violent scene would erupt. He took this strategy to all aspects of his life and whenever he heard adults raise their voices he froze and imagined himself as wallpaper. Jane, aged five, described her strategy when her father or grandfather was sexually abusing her. 'When the monsters came, I pretended I was Supergirl and flew round the room but I only did it when the monsters came.'

Traumatic events may be time limited or ongoing. Time-limited traumatic events include road accidents, natural disasters and assaults. These events may have many traumatic moments. Survivors of the New Orleans hurricane disaster, for example, will have experienced multiple traumas as the events progressed.

Sammi, aged 11, lived in Africa for the first six years of his life. When he was five, he remembered his mother being assaulted in front of family members by soldiers of a rebel army and now, four years later, when he heard crying and shouting it made him extremely fearful. He had placed all his special possessions from Africa in a locked suitcase which he kept with him whenever possible. The suitcase became a kind of talisman connecting him with his past, the people, places and events which shaped his life experiences. He was able to settle with his foster carers in England by keeping his past locked in his suitcase. When he felt safe and secure he was able to talk to his carer and show her his possessions from his past. It was important for him to control the opening and closing of the suitcase so that nobody else had access to his memories unless he chose to show them. The key to the suitcase was his most prized possession and it somehow linked his past to his present.

Ongoing traumatic events include chronic domestic violence, physical and sexual abuse, community violence and war. Tommy, aged eight, invented the following story, which was his imaginary version of a police raid at his family home, and he combined his story with police dramas from TV. He had lived in fear of violence and abuse for the first four years of his life as his mother's addiction to heroin and other hard drugs left her incapable of protecting her children from her violent acquaintances. The police had raided his family home on several occasions and he had been frightened by the shouting and screaming as the police searched his house. Now Tommy was with new parents who wanted to adopt him so he felt able to play.

The Police Investigation

Two cars crash so the fire engine comes.
A third car crashes.
They are having an argument about who would get the drugs.
The three cars got away.
The police are out looking for them.
There were five police cars.

Two of them were hiding.
They had a huge search.
Loads of fire brigades.
The police came straight out of the station.
They said they were looking for drug dealers.
You must know the code to get in there.
Every police officer is looking for them.
They had bazooka guns.
The army on one side,
The police and fire brigade on the other.
They had Landrovers.
They saw the police were about to move.
They fired their guns.
The army came in.
Helicopters, cannons everything.
It was chock-a-block.
The soldiers moved in different places.
They fired at the drug dealers' cars.
But the cars quickly moved about.
Then the cars were surrounded.
There was a huge group of police and army.
So the dealers gave up.
The dealers got out of the cars.

At times Tommy had intrusive thoughts about events from his early years and he became restless and tense. He enjoyed making stories which included aspects of his lived experiences. Repetition in his stories was important although each storyline was expanded during a retelling. These explorations seemed to offer him some control over his fears. After story-making he liked to relax with slime or Play Doh and this sensory play helped him regulate his emotional responses to past memories.

He was beginning to feel safe with his new family, although he tested their intentions by resisting their warm and loving approaches. However, at bedtime Tommy started to relax, so his parents initiated 'soothing sessions' when they sang to him or read a story. He was still afraid of warm physical contact but was soothed by singing and reading. After the sessions he was able to initiate a warm hug to his father or mother, whoever was with him.

Tommy spoke to me about his resistance to accepting his new circumstances, that he didn't want to 'give in'. 'Life's a bitch,' he said and we would laugh together. Perhaps we adults minimize how infuriating it is for a child to be placed in a strange family, however warm and kindly, however well prepared. We all feel anxiety when we move to a new place but to move in with strange adults is an enormous challenge for the child who doesn't trust adults to care for him.

Reactions to post-traumatic stress

The core symptoms can be described in three categories: hyperarousal/hypervigilance, intrusion and constriction (Van der Kolk, Van der Hart and Marmar 1996).

- *Hyperarousal* is where there is a persistent expectation of danger and all threatening situations are reacted to as if part of the original life-threatening event.

- *Hypervigilance* is characterized by an exaggerated startle reaction, for example a jumpiness in the face of normal sounds. This creates high levels of fear, anxiety and tension, leading to an inability to control emotional responses. The anxiety and fear can lead to insomnia, irritability and impaired concentration for non-trauma-related activity.

Hyperarousal and hypervigilance means that the child remains alerted to danger and ready for flight.

- *Intrusion* arises from the difficulty in integrating the emotions related to the traumatic events. Images in the form of flashbacks or nightmares, somatic experiences and other anxiety reactions are triggered by situations which might resemble the original trauma. For example, Jane was still afraid at night in her adoptive home when she heard footsteps as the adults came to bed. She often had nightmares followed by pains in her stomach.

- *Constriction* mirrors the numbing response which the trauma created and leads to the active avoidance of any situation which might evoke trauma-related emotions and can become a generalized detachment from everyday situations which require any kind of emotional response.

Traumatized children feel the world is a frightening place and find it hard to trust anyone, especially adults who have a caring role.

The narrative focus to help traumatized children

White (2005) holds that the primary focus of a narrative approach is people's expressions of their experiences of life. The narrative expressions of both adults and children act as interpretations and through these interpretations people give meaning to their experiences of life, which seem sensible to themselves and to others. He states that meaning does not pre-exist the interpretation of experience. He considers that expressions are constitutive of life, the world that is lived through; they structure experience and inform future understanding. Expressions have a cultural context and are informed by the knowledge and practices of life that are culturally determined. The structure of narrative provides the principal frame of intelligibility for people in their day-to-day lives. It is through this frame that people link together the events of life in sequences that unfold through time according to specific themes.

It is important for children who have experienced trauma to have a narrative of events which makes sense of their experience to their own satisfaction. Young children often make a fiction from their traumatic memories but there is always a connection to their lived trauma. David, aged six, had lived for five years with his mother, who had mental health problems and experienced psychotic episodes in his presence, which frightened and traumatized him. He developed narratives about a witch and he was able to express his fear and anger through these fictions.

The Witch

There was once a witch who had purple nails, long fingers, a magic cat and a broomstick. She made spells by muttering and shouting and when she made spells she made her broomstick fly.

She was very bad and turned people into stone. They died. Just children.

Before the children died they said: 'You are a bully, a bastard, a shit head, a dick, a mean bitch. I hope you rot in hell.'

The witch laughed. 'Just die,' she said.

Then somebody came along who nobody knows and killed the witch. He set the children free and alive again. When they grow up they always had a remember of that witch.

Traumatized children in a new family

Children who come to live in a family who want to foster or adopt them come with a story about themselves and their life as it has been experienced. Like Tommy they might understand parents as violent abusing people who terrorize each other and hurt children. Like David they might think their new mother is a witch. They might understand the role of the father as the man who comes to their room late at night to touch and tickle which is nice but scary, or the mother who is so 'out of it' on drugs that there is nothing to eat and the house is cold.

The baggage of hurt goes with the child to their new home and the struggle is for the new family to understand and help the child trust enough to begin to find a place in the family. A playing relationship between the child and carers can bond them towards becoming a family group. Together, through pretend play, they can explore helpful stories and unhelpful stories about what parents can do and what children can become in a loving family, and what the family might want to change and what they need to keep as their history develops together. When working with families who are seeking to find ways to attach to each other it is important for the therapist or professional worker to facilitate this process by helping both parents and child to negotiate and speak together about the meanings and understanding they have of family life.

The adoptive parents have a story about the life experiences of the child they wish to adopt. They are desperate to take away the pain and hurt of a traumatic past. One way for parents/carers to understand how their child might be feeling is for them to make up a story using the toys in the way the child has played or perhaps to draw a picture using the same theme as the child has drawn. So Mary's story in the Introduction was played out by her with her parents listening. This gave her carers an insight into her mistrust and anger at the way adults behave when they are drinking. Remember the story:

Once upon a time there was a wicked witch and a wicked dragon. They lived together.

They put the birdie in the cage.
They hurt the birdie and hit it.
They drank a lot.
They hurt the dog and the baby.
The wicked witch is dead.
Mary killed her.
She put the animals in the cage and shot the animals.
They are all dead.

Mary instructed her parents how to place the toys to make the story. She was in command. Her parents placed the toys as she instructed. They felt her mistrust as they narrated her story back to her using the toys and the environments Mary had made. Mary felt they had validated her experience and was proud that they wanted to play it. After sharing this event together, Mary skipped out of the room into the garden onto the swing and we could hear her singing as she flew higher and higher. Her parents were saddened by their recreation of the play but had more understanding of her perceptions of the world. They also realized that in playing Mary had relieved some of her burden, leaving her to enjoy singing and swinging in the garden. She was beginning to trust her parents with her history and this left her free to explore the world about her.

The death of a parent: John's story

John was 11 years old. He lived with his younger sister and his adoptive parents. For his first four years John had lived with his birth mother. She neglected John due to her misuse of alcohol. John and his sister were then placed in foster care for four years. They were very attached to their foster carers. A year after being placed with his adoptive family, John's birth mother died, then a year later his foster mother was killed in a car accident. John was devastated and the family were finding it difficult to manage his behaviour. John stuck to his adoptive mother like glue, constantly invading her personal space. He was unable to concentrate and found it difficult to make friends at school. He found it difficult to understand what was required for appropriate social interaction. His younger sister coped better than John and was able to confide in her parents and friends in ways which John couldn't manage. She was very loving and supportive of John which helped him.

We worked together to help John. I did some individual play with him, then sessions with John and his sister, then play sessions with the whole family. John's mother also decided to have her own counselling because she felt that memories of her own childhood were interfering with her relationship with the children. John and I began with narratives of his life as he saw it. There had been difficult times with his birth mother, but a good memory of happy times with his foster family. The death of his birth mother and foster mother were both devastating events. He was desperate for friends, to be able to share happy times. He felt helpless but he wanted to be clever, funny and weird.

The family worked with John to support him in his social interactions with others, helping him when he felt desperate with calming techniques through music and breathing exercises. We enjoyed sharing his quirky sense of humour. He loved Ricky Gervais's *Flanimals*. All family members defined themselves as one of the 'flanimals' and this freed them to say negative things as well as positive without others feeling personally criticized. It was just fun becoming a 'flanimal'.

John was able to talk about his sadness and fear created by the loss of his 'mothers'. Would this happen again? Do all mothers die? Unbearable pain at times made him jumpy, no wonder he kept so close to his adoptive mother. But he had a natural optimism, loved his adoptive parents and appreciated his sister's care. Through her own counselling his mother was able to recover her warmth of feeling for John, who was beginning to find friends with the support of his parents and sister. There are still good days and bad days but the family can talk together and be supportive to each other, finding ways to solve problems as they arise.

John liked the story of *The Mermaid of Kessock*, which in many ways mirrored his own feelings of abandonment

The Mermaid of Kessock

A man named Paterson was once walking along the shore near Kessock Ferry when he saw, sitting on the dark misty deep, a mermaid, who he tried to detain by wading into the water and pulling some of the scales from her tail, in obedience to the old belief that, if even part of her fishtail was removed, a mermaid was compelled to assume human form.

Before his eyes the transformation took place, and the sea-maiden stood up before him, tall and fair. She had long silky hair that was as yellow as gold and soft as the curling foam of the sea; her eyes were wide and clear and blue as the sky; her lips were as red as winter berries and as tempting as fruits of summer; and in place of the fish tail she had slim white feet.

Paterson fell desperately in love with the sea-maiden and took her home as his bride. The scales he carefully hid in an outhouse.

He lived in a cottage by the shore and the raging noise of the waves, which sounded night and day at the foot of the cottage garden, filled his mermaid bride with longing to return to her home to the land under the waves where she had been nursed by the ocean and rocked by the storms.

She used to plead with her husband to let her go, promising that if he did so their family would always be blessed with a plentiful supply of fish and that no members of it would ever be drowned at Kessock Ferry, but he refused.

One day one of the children discovered the scales in the outhouse and took them to his mother, who straightaway made for the shore and became a mermaid again.

Not since that day has the mermaid of Kessock been seen; but there are still local people who firmly believe in her existence, and declare that she still watches over her descendants and keeps them from peril at sea.

We talked about how lost the mermaid must feel being forced to live in a strange world. How Paterson her husband bullied her. Although she had children with Paterson she was desperate to return to her own kingdom under the sea. And we talked about how the child who discovered her scales in the outhouse must feel about being the one who gave his mother her freedom but also lost her in the process. We played around with the story. John dictated a letter to me as though he was the mermaid writing home to her family under the sea. Then another letter, as though he was the child who had found the scales and in so doing had lost his mother to the sea kingdom. We imagined what they might say to each other if they met many years later. John said that it was comforting to know that the mermaid watches over her family and we imagined what his two mothers might say to him and how they would want him to be happy.

I told John the Russian story of *The Three Daughters*, which he found very soothing.

The Three Daughters

Once upon a time there lived a woman. She worked all day and night to feed and clothe her daughters. And the three daughters grew up swift as swallows and with faces that resembled bright moons. One after another they married and went away.

Many years went by. The old woman became very ill and sent a red squirrel to her daughters. 'Tell them to come quickly to me, little friend.'

'Oi,' said the eldest when she heard the sad news from the squirrel. 'I should be glad to go but I've got to clean these two basins first.'

'Clean two basins,' said the squirrel, angrily, 'then may you never be parted from them.' And the basins suddenly jumped up from the table and caught hold of the daughter from above and below. She fell to the floor and crawled out of the house in the shape of a big tortoise.

The squirrel tapped on the door of the second daughter. 'Oi,' she responded. 'I'd run to my mother at once but I'm very busy. I have to weave some cloth for the fair.'

'Well now, weave for the whole of your life without stopping,' said the squirrel. And the second daughter was turned into a spider.

The youngest daughter was kneading dough when the squirrel knocked. The daughter did not say a word and without even wiping her hands she ran to her mother.

'Always bring sweetness and joy to people, my dear child,' the squirrel said to her, 'and people will love and cherish you and your children, and grandchildren and great grandchildren.'

And indeed the youngest daughter lived a great many years and everybody loved her. And when the time came for her to die she turned into a golden bee.

The whole day long all through the summer the bee gathers honey for people and its front paws are always covered with sweet pollen and in the winter when everything is dying from the cold the little bee sleeps in a warm hive and when it wakes up it will eat honey and sugar.

John defined this as a soothing story because he liked the repetition and the squirrel's responses to the sisters. There are kind and unkind sisters as well as kind and unkind mothers. The end was very soothing for him as he thought of the bee covered in pollen.

Overcoming a specific trauma: Peter's story

Some children may have experienced a specific trauma which has subsequently disturbed the family dynamic and the therapist can explore with the child and carers how to shift some of the stress and find new ways of coping in the family. Peter was six when I met him. His parents were separated, but in a fit of anger and despair, his father had come to the house, taken Peter and his mother and kept them hostage for three days. During that time he had assaulted Peter's mother and threatened both of them with a gun. He was subsequently arrested by the police and was now in prison.

I saw the family for the first time some weeks after the event because mother and son were finding it difficult to settle after such a shocking incident. Peter's mother took out her anger on Peter and he felt blamed and responsible for his father's behaviour. He felt he should have rescued his mother and protected her from his father's violence. During my talks with Peter's mother when she felt angry with him, I told her the story of *The Missing Axe*.

The Missing Axe

A man whose axe was missing suspected his neighbour's son. The boy looked like a thief, walked like a thief, spoke like a thief.

But the man found his axe while digging in the valley and the next day he saw his neighbour's son. The boy walked, looked and spoke like any other child.

We began to talk about Peter as a small child threatened by his father with a gun and how Peter's mother had felt trying to protect both of them. She started to think of him as he was, a small child, not an adult who should have protected her.

Peter began to talk about the incident and we were able to work out together what was possible in such circumstances and what was not possible, due to his father being bigger and stronger and holding a gun. Peter said that he had jumped on his father's back several times to try to stop him. He repeated this often, seeking confirmation that he had done his best. In play Peter evolved a story about Peter Pan and Captain Hook. I was Captain Hook and he was Peter Pan. We both had swords and were fighting together but, although Captain Hook was bigger and stronger, Peter Pan was quicker and agile and managed to outwit Captain Hook and win the fight.

We played this scene many times throughout our meetings and as Captain Hook I admired Peter Pan's agility and ability to outwit the Captain. This play was helpful to Peter. It was a wish fulfilled in play if not in the reality event and gave Peter a sense of power and control which he had not experienced when his father was so violent. But he was able to think positively about what he had actually managed by jumping on his father's back and trying to stop him hurting his mother. He became reconciled that he had done what he could. It was only after the play that Peter was able to describe what had happened in reality. Some children do not wish to talk about the reality experience but stay in the play they have made and we co-construct solutions together within the play.

I spoke with Peter's mother about his feelings of helplessness and she also began to think about what Peter had done and how frightening it must have been for him. She began to talk to Peter about his bravery in jumping on his father's back. They began to watch the video of Peter Pan together and Peter told her of our Peter Pan story. They began to play together and she remembered the story of the three musketeers, 'One for all, and all for one.' They played the two musketeers and both mother and son felt more powerful as they played together, us against the world. Laughter returned to the house. The memories of the violence still lurked in the dark places and the uncertain times but the bond between mother and son remained strong with the acceptance that they had both done their best.

Adults can support children who have experienced trauma in their lives by first acknowledging what has happened and not minimizing the pain. It is important not to force children to talk about their fears if they do not wish to do so. Children will often solve their anxieties through a pretend story rather than talk about their reality world. It is important to find time to soothe children, finding out what calms them down. Many children enjoy music, others like an adult to read them a story and some like help with relaxation and breathing techniques.

A soothing programme

Jane, aged 14, learnt to soothe herself. Every day after school she went to the sitting room on her own. She played her favourite music very loudly and danced until exhausted. Then she changed the tempo of the music to a slower beat with a dreamy quality. She then lay full length on the floor and felt the tension flow from her body until she relaxed. Her mother had worried about this activity but was reassured as Jane said it helped her after the stress of the school day. We added some breathing exercises as she lay on the floor to assist the relaxation. Jane enjoyed this personal time more and more as she was supported and respected by her mother for so imaginatively learning to manage her own feelings.

For younger children after energetic exercise, perhaps to music or on a trampoline, a story, then breathing exercises, then another story can create a soothing ritual which can become part of the family life, perhaps daily or once or twice a week depending on the needs of the child and the family. The following two stories and breathing exercises can perhaps be a template for a similar family activity. First, a cheery story.

Tiddalik

Once upon a time there was a frog called Tiddalik.
He was the biggest frog in the entire world.
He was very, very fat.
He was the most unhappy and miserable frog in the whole world.
He spent his time hiding under huge rocks.
It was dark and wet there.
All day, every day he sat under the rocks.
Frowning, frowning, frowning.
One day Tiddalik became very thirsty and he drank an entire lake dry.
Still he was thirsty.
So he moved to a river and drank that dry.
Still he was thirsty.

So he went from place to place drinking every lake and river dry.
Soon he had drunk every drop of water in the entire country.
The grass shrivelled, the trees and flowers died and the soil crumbled.
The other creatures feared for their lives, thinking they would die of thirst.
But a wise old wombat came up with the answer.
'We must make Tiddalik laugh. Then the muscles in his belly will contract and all the water will burst out of his mouth.'
So the animals tried to make Tiddalik laugh.
First the kangaroo tried dancing on her tail with koala bears balancing on her head.
No laughter came.
Then a duck-billed platypus told a joke.
Bad joke, not funny.
Everybody had a go.
Including a dingo, a kiwi, bush baby, ostrich, crocodile, parrots of all kinds.
No laughter came.
The frog was gloomy.
He sat under rocks, looking miserable and the earth got drier and drier.
Then Nabunum the eel came along and began to tie himself in knots.
A result.
First Tiddalik's face twitched, his eyes twinkled.
Then, when the eel tried to belly dance, Tiddalik burst into a huge roar of laughter.
Sure enough, as wombat had predicted, the water poured out of the frog's mouth and all the lakes and river flowed with water, and the land became fertile again.

Then some breathing exercises:

1. *Deep breathing.* Lie on the floor. Place each hand at the base of the ribs, left hand to left side, right hand to right side. Breathe in through the nose to a silent count of three. Hold the breath for a silent count of three. Then breathe out to a silent count of three.

2. *Yawning and sighing.* Lie on the floor on your back and give an enormous silent yawn. Then yawn and, as you breathe out, let

a quiet sound come out. Then yawn and let a sigh come out. Then yawn and let a soothing sound come out.

3.   *Humming.* Breathe in deeply. Then start to hum. Quietly at first, then a little louder, then quietly again until you feel relaxed.

4.   *Visualization: Cocooned in the shell.* Lie on the floor on your back and give an enormous silent yawn. Then curl up on the floor like a snail. Close your eyes and keep them closed. Imagine that you are in a cocoon surrounded by a soft strong shell that protects you. Imagine what it is like inside the cocoon. How much space is there? Can you move around? Very slowly break out of the cocoon. When you break out stretch yourself and as you stretch make a long sigh.

End with a story, a way to share the soothing for storyteller and listener.

The Fly: A Story from Vietnam

Everyone in the village knew the moneylender, he was rich and smart. He made lots of money then retired to a beautiful house with a magnificent garden. But he still went on lending money because he couldn't resist the power that his money gave him and the power he had over the people who were in debt to him.

One day he went to visit a poor family who couldn't pay him the money they owed. He was going to take some of the poor family's possessions if they couldn't pay him. When he got to the poor man's house the only person there was a young boy of eight playing in the dirt yard.

'Are your parents home?' asked the moneylender.

'No sir,' said the boy.

'Well, then, where are they?'

The little boy went on playing and did not answer.

The moneylender asked again, 'Where are your parents?'

Slowly the boy answered, 'Well, sir, my father has gone to cut down trees and plant dead ones and my mother is at the market place selling the wind and buying the moon.'

'What are you talking about?' shouted the moneylender. 'Tell me where they are or I will beat you with my stick.'

The boy repeated his answer.

'Listen, little devil,' shouted the moneylender. 'If you tell me where they really are and what they are doing I will forget all about the money your parents owe me.'

'Why are you joking with me?' asked the boy. 'Do you expect me to believe what you are saying?'

'Well, there is heaven and there is earth to witness my promise,' said the moneylender.

The boy laughed. 'Sir, heaven and earth cannot talk and therefore cannot testify. I want some living thing to be our witness.'

Catching sight of a fly alighting on a nearby bamboo pole the moneylender said, 'There is a fly, he can be our witness.'

Looking at the fly on the pole the boy said, 'A fly is good enough witness for me. Well, sir, here it is. My father has gone to cut down bamboo and make a fence with them for a man by the river. And my mother has gone to the market to sell fans to buy oil for our lamps. Isn't that what you would call selling the wind to buy the moon?'

Shaking his head, the moneylender had to admit that the boy was a clever one. However, he thought he could still trick the child as he didn't believe a fly could be a witness to anyone. He said goodbye to the boy promising that he would return to make good his promise.

After a few days the moneylender returned. The child's parents were at home because it was late in the day. A nasty scene followed with the moneylender demanding payment of the debt. The couple pleaded with the moneylender to give them more time to pay him, but he refused. The moneylender was shouting and the parents were pleading. This argument woke the little boy who had been sleeping.

He ran to his father saying, 'Father, you don't have to pay your debt. This gentleman promised he would forget all about the money you owed him.'

'Nonsense,' said the moneylender, shaking his stick at father and son. 'Are you going to listen to the child's fairy story? I never spoke a word to this boy. Now are you going to pay or not?'

The whole affair ended by being brought before the mandarin who ruled the country.

Not knowing what to believe the poor parents brought their son to the court. Their son's insistence about the moneylender's promise was their only encouragement. The mandarin began by asking the boy to tell exactly what had happened between himself and the moneylender. The boy told the mandarin all the explanations he gave to the moneylender in exchange for the debt.

'Well,' the mandarin said to the boy, 'if this man here has made such a promise to you, we have only your word for it. How do we know that you have not invented the whole story yourself? In a case such as this we need a witness to vouch for what happened and you have none.'

The boy remained calm and said that naturally there was a witness to their conversation.

'Who is that, child?' the mandarin asked.

'A fly your honour.'

'A fly, what do you mean, a fly? Watch out young man, fantasies are not to be tolerated in this place.' The mandarin looked angry and his face became stern.

'Yes your honour, a fly. A fly which was alighting on this gentleman's nose.'

The boy leapt from his seat.

'Insolent little devil, that's a pack of lies,' screamed the moneylender. The moneylender roared and his face became purple with rage. 'The fly was not on my nose. He was on the house pole...' but he stopped dead.

It was, however, too late.

The majestic mandarin burst out laughing. He could not help himself. Then the whole court burst out laughing. The boy's parents laughed although rather timidly. And the boy and the moneylender also laughed.

With one hand on his stomach the mandarin waved the other hand towards the moneylender. 'Now, now that's all settled. You have indeed made your promises to the child. House pole or no house pole, your conversation did happen after all. The court says you must keep your promise.'

And still laughing he dismissed all parties.

CHAPTER 4

Making My World
Being in a Family

Baby Janet

This baby called Janet is six months old.
She lives with her gran, mum and step-dad.
He doesn't live with them all the time.
He left when she was born
because he didn't like her
because she was a girl and not a boy.
Mother felt sad and mother and grandmother
decided to bring up Janet together.
Janet is in the bedroom.
It is night time.
The baby feels safe.
The baby is sad because the mother is sad.
She should have been a boy.
The baby might be sad or not.
She doesn't know what to say.
She doesn't think about it.
She is angry with dad.

Sarah is five and lives with her mother and grandmother. She never knew her father and her step-father left soon after she was born. Sarah's pretend story about Janet mirrors her own understanding of herself and the sense of responsibility she feels for her mother's sadness. Her identity is compromised by the thought that she is to blame for being a girl and that, if she had been a boy, her step-father would have stayed with the family and her mother would be happy. This is her dominant story. She has taken responsibility for the adults' behaviour and feelings and considers herself unlovable.

John, aged seven, was desperate for nurture from his mother. Both parents lived together but John's mother constantly denigrated men. John thought that if he was like a girl then his mother would like him better but she continued to criticize him for being like a girl. Catch 22: be a boy and I will hate you, be a girl and I will despise you. John was emotionally abused by this family narrative and his mother found it difficult to change her views.

Sarah's mother and grandmother understood her family story which did not accurately describe their circumstances. They played together and used her pretend stories as a basis for questions and conversations about 'Janet' and her ideas about herself and her family. Together they restructured the stories to show that it was the adults who were making decisions about being together or not being together and that it had nothing to do with 'Janet' being a girl baby. They cemented their family relationship by being three females together taking pride in their gender. Play and questioning ideas rather than 'telling' a child they are wrong is more helpful in changing distorted thinking. After time, Sarah developed a secure attachment to her mother and grandmother but John's mother was unable to shift her position and her ambivalent feelings about men.

It is important for families who adopt or foster children and for families whose children have a limited understanding of social interaction to have some knowledge of attachment theory, because their children may have struggles to achieve trusting relationships both inside and outside the family. They might need special support and more explanations about the meanings of interactions with others in their social world.

Attachment theory

The two major attachment theorists, Bowlby (1969–80) and Ainsworth (Ainsworth *et al.* 1978), argued that secure attachments in the early years are central to the development of social competence and insecure attachments create difficulties in relationships and problems in later development. Attachment is an inborn system of the brain that evolved to keep the child safe. It enables the child to seek proximity to the parent/carer, go to the parent/carer in time of distress for comfort and internalize the relationship with the parent/carer as an internal model of a secure base. The sense of security is built on repeated experiences of connection with the attachment figure. In secure attachments the infant uses the caregiver as a secure base from which to explore the environment. In insecure attachments the infant either avoids the caregiver or shows resistance or ambivalence in their relationship with the caregiver.

Ainsworth and colleagues (1978) described three principal patterns of attachment:

1. *Secure attachment* is when the person is confident that her parent or parent figure will be available, responsive and helpful when he or she encounters difficult or frightening situations. With this assurance, he or she can explore the world. The parent, especially the mother, promotes this confidence by being readily available – sensitive to her child's signals, and lovingly responsive when he or she seeks comfort.

2. *Insecure anxious resistant attachment* is when the person is uncertain whether the parent will be available, responsive or helpful when called upon. Because of the uncertainty, the person is always prone to separation anxiety, tends to cling, and is anxious about exploring the world. The parent promotes the pattern by being unpredictable to some extent: sometimes available and helpful, but not at other times. The pattern is shown by persons who have been separated from the parent, and also by parents who threaten abandonment as a means of control.

3. *Insecure anxious avoidant attachment* is when the person has no confidence that they will be comforted when seeking care; on the contrary, they expect a rebuff. When such a person tries to live life without the love and support of others, he or she tries to become emotionally self-sufficient and may become self-absorbed in ways that damage social relationships with others.

These three categories of attachment were further extended by the work of Main (1991) to include a fourth category:

4.   *Insecure disorganized disorientated attachment* is when the person
      has an unusually high level of fear and might be disorientated.
      This can result from experiences of abuse by adults or the
      death of parents or caregivers.

Many children who come into care have experienced insecure attachments and develop a view of themselves as unlovable and not worthy of
love and affection. Their pretend play and narratives are often about scary
places where people have to fend for themselves. James, aged seven, experienced families and the world as scary. He told many stories about scary
places with individuals fighting monsters. His stories usually end with a
yearning for a safe place to live, but always alone.

The Scary Magic Place

This is a magic place.
It is scary magic.
It is a beach and the sea.
Lots of layers of sand.
There are two seas.
The dragons are waiting for the tide to come in.
They are scary.
They roar and eat you up.
They have no teeth.
They suck you up with their tonsils.
There is a knight called Sir Edward.
He wants to kill the dragons
Because all his army is killed by them.
He is going to risk his life.
Because all his army are dead,
And his parents died in the war.
He has killed one dragon with a sword and a spear.
There is a snake who lives with the dragons.
They have reunited.
'I want to eat a human,' said the snake.
The dragons are killed by the knight.
He goes away.
The land is being made into a beach
By Sir Edward.
He is building a castle to live in.
He miniscules himself so he can go through.
The End.

James also felt that he was part of this chaotic world and he was afraid would fail when he went to live with his adoptive parents. He made another story with the slime about himself:

> There was once a boy
> Who was dripping thick red blood
> Because he felt like it.
> He touched his skin and it just began to bleed.
> Because he had a problem with his skin.
> He liked to see the blood drip
> But not too much.

This kind of self-loathing and a lack of understanding about family life can be very frightening for new parents. Sometimes the needs of the children feed into the parents' own anxiety and the struggles they might have with their own family history and this difficulty can influence the way they perceive family life. There is an ongoing research project which began in 1995, 'The Adoption and Attachment Representations Study' (Anna Freud Centre n.d.) which is investigating the development of attachment relationships in children who were previously maltreated and have recently been adopted. One of the measures used in the study is the Adult Attachment Interview which was developed by Mary Main and her colleagues at Berkeley University (George, Kaplan and Main 1985). This interview has been shown to be a reliable and valid measure of the degree to which adults have 'come to terms' with their childhood history. How adults think and feel about their own experiences of parent–child relationships during their own childhood is strongly related to the quality of the attachment relationship which develops with their own children.

Adult narratives of childhood attachments

Adult narratives of childhood have been codified. The following list sums up Steele's (2002) description of four patterns of attachment defined in the Adult Attachment Interview:

1. *Dismissing.* You were parentally rejected or neglected during childhood but this is only mentioned indirectly. You work hard to protect your unrealistically positive or normalized

image of your parents and your childhood. You tend to dismiss or devalue the significance of childhood attachment relationships.

2.   *Autonomous.* You were well loved and supported by your parents during childhood and/or experienced adversity and perhaps severe pain. You understand the past and its influence on the present. Yours is a coherent, credible narrative that conveys a strong valuing of attachment.

3.   *Preoccupied.* You had many caregiving duties towards your parents during childhood, such that roles were frequently reversed with your attachment needs being compromised. You are angry and confused about these experiences but you value attachments. The task of narrating your experiences is rather painful.

4.   *Unresolved.* You have suffered loss and trauma in childhood or adulthood and you are still grieving. You feel responsible in some way for the loss or trauma and you don't see that as unreasonable on your part. The loss or trauma does not yet belong to your past.

Sometimes when children are experiencing difficulties socially, it is easy to demonize them as though they live in isolation. We are inclined to forget the role played by others in the children's interactions. This is not helpful because we can't evaluate an interaction without exploring how people interact together and so we are unable to learn what went wrong with a view to putting it right in the future.

Although initially James presented very frightening thoughts and feelings to his adoptive family they coped with his fears and were able to explore the impact of his lack of ability to attach on their own past experiences with their parents. It was a long struggle but gradually James realized that his parents were not going to give up on him and he learnt to value himself. He is still impulsive, still finding social interaction confusing, but knows that he has parents who accept him as he is and don't pressurize him to make a relationship with them which would overwhelm him.

Helping children who struggle with attachments

Children who have been maltreated, abused or neglected can lose their capacity to trust adults to care for them. Sroufe (1995) states that infants are not capable of regulating their own emotions and arousal and need the assistance of their caregiver in this process. How the infant learns to regulate his or her emotions will depend heavily on how the caregiver regulates his or her own emotions. As children become better at express-ing their needs and emotions they learn self-regulating skills. This is not a one-way process. As the caregiver affects the infant so the infant affects the caregiver. Stern (1985) defines this as attunement; that is, when the caregiver is sensitive to the verbal and non-verbal cues of the child and is able to put himself or herself into the mind of the child.

Harris (1994) says that in the course of the first year the infant under-stands three major components of human emotion. First, a person's emotional expression has a meaningful content with implications for one's own current emotional state. Second, other people are, under normal circumstances, responsive to the emotional state of the self. Third, other people's emotions are typically directed at an intentional target, a person, location or object in the immediate environment, which means that another person's emotion can have an implication for one's own emotion with respect to that target.

Research on attachment theory has focused on the sensitivity of the carer and how that might impact on the emotional communication of the child, so children of depressed mothers show a 'depressed' style when with their mothers and also with strangers (Field et al. 1988). Harris (1994) holds that expressions of anger create a disturbing state for infants and young children. They frequently elicit a tense, frozen attention, which temporarily suppresses any other ongoing activity. Children's responses to sustained exposure to anger can for some serve as a licence to engage in hostile behaviour, for others it arouses solicitous concern and others attempt to screen it out.

Children who take on the adult role

Many children from unsafe families decide that as adults cannot be trusted they must parent themselves and if they have younger siblings then they must parent them as well. In many ways this can be a powerful role and when such a sibling group moves to a new family then the child-mother can challenge the adult mother wanting to take her role. I remember a small eight-year-old girl fighting with her adoptive mother in the kitchen, challenging the adult as she cooked a meal. It can take time and sensitive support to give such a child permission to enjoy being a child rather than taking on the responsibility of parenting her siblings. Adolescent girls often have difficulties with their friends as they feel they must be responsible for everybody being happy and getting it together, and in the course of the in-fighting and jealousy engendered in the group it is often the 'mothering' adolescent who bears the brunt of the group hostility.

Such children do have a yearning to be nurtured by their parents. Belle, aged five, played the following story:

> Once upon a time there was a very cross crocodile.
> He smashed his teeth together shouting, 'I want my mum.'
> Mum said, 'What are you doing?'
> The crocodile said, 'What are you doing here, Mum? What are you doing on the rock?'
> Mum said, 'I've just come for a wee play.'
> Today Mum is being sensible.
> She is not being drunk.
> So she could look after crocodile.
> She could.

Belle is in a supportive foster placement waiting for an adoptive family; she has been in care for two years. She has a younger brother and she protects him and mothers him. He finds it difficult to do anything without her permission but it is 'us against the world'. This is her story about her and her brother:

> Once upon a time there was a big red pond.
> It was a good happy place.
> Belle and Sandy live there.
> They lived on their own.
> No mummy and daddy.
> Just Belle and Sandy.
> Daddy told Belle she had to look after Sandy.
> They are happy on their own.

They played and played and jumped in the big pond.
There was a crocodile in the pond.
It played with Belle and Sandy.
There was a small jelly hand in the pond.
Belle put her hand in the pond.
It felt nice and soft.

I sometimes tell children the story *The Eye Cannot Deceive.* We can talk about Tortoise who mistrusts his mother and wants to control everything and how in this story Tortoise is wrong about his mother. The stories I tell don't exactly mirror the children's life experiences but there is enough of a similarity for the children to feel that their issues are not just their own but have been experienced and understood by others.

The Eye Cannot Deceive

At one time Tortoise lived with his mother. He did not like this very much because his mother often got angry and shouted at him. Besides she was a fat old lady and ate a great deal, so Tortoise had to work very hard to find enough food for both of them.

One day tortoise went to the farm and collected seven baskets of green vegetables. He carried the baskets home to his mother and said: 'Mammy, I'd like you to cook these vegetables at once because I am very hungry.'

Mammy Tortoise began to cook the greens, and when she had prepared them she put them back in the baskets and they fitted easily into three.

Tortoise came in, sat down, looked at the three baskets on the table and said: 'Bring the other four baskets of vegetables in. Didn't you hear me say that I'm hungry?'

'What other vegetables?' his mother answered, 'That's all there was.'

Tortoise was furious. He felt sure that his mother had eaten the food in the other baskets. He shouted at her and when she started to get angry he pushed her out of the house and told her never to return.

Tortoise sat down and ate his meal. He thought, 'I'm glad she's gone. Now she won't ever be able to eat my food again.'

When he had finished eating he still felt very hungry, so he went to the farm again and filled his seven baskets of food for the second time.

He cooked the vegetables and began to put them into his baskets again. He looked in the pot. He counted the baskets, there were three, and then he realized that he had sent away his mother for no reason.

When he thought about what he had done he felt sad.

Children who feel alone in the world

Many children who have been unnurtured and children who have a literal understanding of their social world often feel alone and isolated from others. They are afraid of affection in case it is impermanent. This is Barry's story.

Stuck in the Slime

Once upon a time there was a big pile of slime and all the people got stuck in the slime, and all the cars. The slime covered everything and the cars and the people couldn't get out of the slime.

The skeleton got stuck and he didn't know what to do. He tried to kick his way out of the slime but he stayed stuck. He swung himself about until he got out in the end. He was happy.

The monster got stuck in the slime and he roared and kicked and got out.

The children got stuck in the slime and they kicked and punched and nodded their heads and shouted 'help!'

The Power Rangers helped them. We don't know if they had parents but they didn't help.

The Power Ranger got stuck. And he kicked, and punched and punched and he done his karate and he got out.

The police even got stuck and tried to drive out, and they got out in the end.

The truck got stuck in the slime. He dried out very quickly.

And all the people meet to go to the messy places and they ran through all the slime and killed it.

And in the end the slime was broken to death.

One more slime to kill.

Now it was the monster's turn. He flew his head in and he banged the slime right in the air and the monster punched him and the slime nearly killed him again. He did his magic head fly. And the monster kicked the slime and punched him far away.

The slime nearly died but it was still alive.

In the end the slime broke.

The slime was dead.

This is a typical story of conflict with each group who have to fight the slime being isolated from each other. There is no interaction or problem solving between the groups. The children have no parents to support them and are another isolated group with no communication or strategies to work together.

John, aged 12, has a narrative about his own birth family which expresses the hurt he feels.

Dave lives in a house, which has a garden with trees. There are three rooms in the house. He lives on his own.

He is a roofer. He likes his home because he built it himself. It has a big garden. He wanted to live on his own.

He has family. He was married with two children. He doesn't know where they are. He spoke to his children when they were little. Now they are teenagers. He is not bothered.

The children feel hurt. The children feel angry.

Dave is a selfish person. He puts his own needs before his family. Dave doesn't really care. He has lots of friends. He goes to the pub. He enjoys that.

Dave is all screwed up. He is selfish to the end.

John has a good understanding of his father and often expresses his own longing for solitude, to live in a place where he can be in control. John says that if you want that kind of life you shouldn't have a family.

I often tell Scottish Broonie stories to these children who can identify with the hardworking creature who is attached to a house or home but is afraid of the people there. My favourite is the Broonie of Blednock. Personally I would like a Broonie to come and live in my house. I talk first about the Broonie as a type of magical creature before telling the story.

The Scottish Broonie is a wild and shaggy creature, usually a small man about 60cm in height. He is wrinkled and brown and wears tattered brown clothes. The Broonies in the Highlands have no fingers or toes; in the Lowlands they have no noses. Most humans are afraid of them because they look so fierce. The Broonie hides in the dark corners of old houses, which he haunts. He watches the comings and goings in the house and at night he cleans the house and does all the tasks which he thinks members of the household might find useful. He is devoted to the family who live in his house and his only purpose is to please them. He doesn't do this for reward but because he is attached to them. Broonies are very touchy creatures and sometimes if family members give him a reward he will take umbrage and leave. He is especially offended by the offer of food, other than a bowl of milk or cream or cake covered with honey, but any other offer of food sends him into paroxysms of rage and hurt. You mustn't pay him, you can thank him but that is all, otherwise he will say farewell and leave never to be seen again. Listen to the story of the Broonie of Blednock.

The Broonie of Blednock

This Broonie had a name although many have no name. He was called Aitken Drum. He lived on a farm and worked hard at night doing all the farm work required. But he always disappeared before sunrise after drinking his bowl of cream left for him by the farmer's wife.

This Broonie had no nose and his mouth was just a gash but he was very hardworking and the farmer was short of workers and needed his services. The neighbours were shocked at the sight of the Broonie but the farmer's wife was wise and realized they had a good bargain, for Aitken Drum could do the work of ten men.

He worked by starlight and by moonlight whenever there was work to be done but he always disappeared before sunrise and nobody saw him drink the cream that was left for him by the farmer's wife.

Aitken Drum stayed at the farm for many years and eventually the children lost their fear of him and loved to listen to his strange unearthly songs and play the Broonie games he taught them when he came to work at twilight.

For many years all went well until one day a foolish young woman thought it was time that Aitken Drum wore clothes and dressed like other folk in the village and left a pair of dirty breeches for him next to the cream left by the farmer's wife. And from that evening he was never seen again.

Only a shepherd passing near a farm one night heard the voice of Aitken Drum crying and grieving because he had been given his fee and could work no more.

And on dark nights when the river is in spate the villagers tremble when they think of the first time they saw Aitken Drum, and children lying in bed at night listening to the wind in the trees think they hear the voice of Aitken Drum singing them to sleep with his mystical song and they long to see him again.

After the storytelling, I often talk with the children about the Broonie, imagining his singing and how soothing that might be. Sometimes we create a Broonie and write to him listing tasks we would like him to complete. We write polite notes with thanks but with not too much affection so the Broonie will accept the communication. We talk about imagining the Broonie singing when the children feel sad or stressed. He is a comforting creature to imagine.

Angry children

Bowlby (1988–90) states that the particular pathways the child proceeds along is determined by the environment he or she meets with, especially the way his or her parents (or parent substitutes) treat him or her and how he or she responds to them. For some children experiencing repeated angry responses from their carers can give the child a licence to behave in similar ways. Some carers actively encourage their children to respond aggressively in their relationships with others. Other children who have not been given help to regulate their emotions are often overwhelmed by their anger and have no means to calm themselves.

Katie, aged seven, explained her confusion living with a new family.

I don't understand the rules.
I don't like shouting.
Even though I get mad
And shout a lot too.
Old dad shouts too much.

Then she drew a picture and told the following story:

> This is daddy's boot.
> He wears it to work.
> He kicks people with it.
> He kicks Big John.
> It hurts when he kicks
> And he goes 'Boo, hoo.'
> The boot is in the house.
> It is a nice house.
> They are having words in the house.
> Big John is crying
> Because he has been kicked.
> There are lots of tears.
> There is another boot.
> It is Big John's boot.
> It is a kicking boot.
> This is a picture of the dark.
> Big John in the dark gets scared.
> He is scared in the dark.
> Little John hates him.

This narrative clearly describes how violence is mirrored from adult to child if it is the only form of communication in the family. Big John can only defend himself by getting a kicking boot like daddy. He holds his boot in the dark, afraid of the dark, fearful of another kicking from daddy. He can only defend himself with his own kicking boot. Violence is this family's only form of communication.

Developing communication systems through play

Play around body awareness and sensory awareness can be helpful because most children who have been a witness to anger and violence in their early years freeze up to stay safe.

Start with breathing exercises.

1. *Attacking fear.* Press your thumbs either side of the nose, below the bones under the eyes. Open your eyes. Breathe deeply. Open your throat. Say 'oh, oh, oh' in a staccato voice.

2. *Forced air.* Suck in air through tightly pursed lips as though sucking on a straw. Push out the air as though squeezing

water from a sponge. Think of the places where your body feels tense.

3. *Drawing me when angry.* We can draw ourselves and colour in the places on our body where we feel anger. What colours can we use to represent anger? Is it the face, teeth grinding, forehead wrinkled? Or the arms and fists, or the stomach all churning up, or the legs? Knees tense, feet ready to kick. So how does this affect us? Can we think sensibly when the body is in this state? What is the difference between being a little bit angry and a big bit angry?

4. *Drawing me when calm.* We can draw ourselves and colour in the places on our body where we feel calm. What is the difference in the body between angry feelings and calm feelings? What is good about both states? What is not good about both states?

Talk together about what makes one angry and explore the different degrees of anger from mild irritation to extreme anger. Find words to express these differences.

I often tell children the following Bengali story about non-violence when we are thinking about degrees of anger.

Non-violence
A very wicked snake infested a road and bit passers-by.

A holy man happened to pass that way and the snake rushed at him to bite him. He calmly looked down at him and said, 'You want to bite me, don't you? Go ahead.'

The snake was subdued by this unusual response and was overpowered by the gentleness of the holy man.

The holy man said, 'Listen, dear friend, how about promising me that you won't bite anyone from now on?'

The snake bowed and nodded agreement.

The holy man went on his way and the snake began its life of innocence and non-violence. Very soon the neighbourhood discovered that the snake was harmless and the boys began to tease it mercilessly. They pelted it with stones and dragged it around by its tail. Still it kept its promise to the holy man and suffered.

Fortunately the holy man happened to come by and see his latest disciple. He was touched by the bruised and battered condition of the snake.

When he asked it what happened the snake said feebly, 'Oh, holy man, you said I should not bite anyone. But people are merciless.'

The holy man answered, 'I asked you not to bite anyone. But I didn't ask you not to hiss.'

Attachment disorders

Some children develop disabling regulatory disorders which Greenspan and Wieder (1993) describe as difficulties in regulating physiological, sensory, attentional and motor or affective processes, and in organizing a calm, alert or affectively positive state. Schore (2003) states that deprivation of early maternal stress modulation is known to trigger not only an exaggerated release of corticosteroids upon exposure to novel experiences but, in addition, inhibitory states that persist for longer periods of time. The result is a quicker access into and a longer duration of dissociated states at later points of stress.

Children with attachment disorders are difficult to parent because they struggle to understand social interaction and feel threatened by adults who try to parent them. *The Diagnostic and Statistical Manual of Mental Disorders* (American Psychiatric Association 1994) describes two types of attachment disorders, 'inhibited' and 'disinhibited'. Inhibited attachment disorder is the persistent failure to initiate and respond to most social interactions in a developmentally appropriate way. Disinhibited attachment disorder is the display of indiscriminate sociability or a lack of selectivity in the choice of attachment figures.

The children's poor impulse control and lack of understanding about other people's feelings can create outbursts of anger. They seek safety, perhaps impulsively attaching to virtual strangers or indulging in 'soothing' behaviours like rocking, biting or picking at their skin. Sometimes the triggers for their outbursts are sensory stimuli which might have been present when the children lived in dangerous environments. Van der Kolk, in his paper 'The body keeps the score' (1994), describes this as the misinterpretation of innocuous stimuli as potential threats.

Family life for these children is a struggle for both the children and their carers. Their mistrust of the adults who care for them means that they test out the relationships again and again. They find it difficult to develop deep emotional bonds and this can be very disheartening for their carers. Adults often get sucked into the children's world view and then they too feel dispirited and helpless. It is very hard not to take the children's behaviour personally. I suggest that carers step back and value the children as they are in the present with all their quirkiness. Adaptation to a new family is a very slow process. The adults have to be predictable, consistent and repetitive. Tasks should be broken down into manageable steps and this will clarify complex multi-step directions. So 'Get your shoes and socks, sit on the stairs and put on your socks then shoes' is far too complex. One task at a time.

The key rule is to avoid power struggles. Children want you to enter their world and get emotionally aroused in the way that they feel for much of the time. So the hour's interrogation about stealing is exhausting for the adults who at the end of the hour might hear the child say how sorry they are but the child interprets this interrogation as their victory because the adults are aroused and have become part of the child's world.

It is better to help the child regulate their emotions by helping them calm down and find a safe place in the house until they feel calm again. Jason, aged eight, had a small tent at the bottom of his bed and when he felt scared he crawled inside and snuggled into a soft blanket. Peter, aged 11, played Elvis Presley on his iPod. Mary, aged four, draws. This is her narrative of her drawing of a snake:

> This is a drawing of a snake.
> He is called Smith [Mary's last name].
> He is a good snake.
> He kisses people because he is a kissing snake.
> He has a nice smile.
> He eats yukky food, yukky water, yukky juice, yukky flies.
> He has no mum and dad
> But Mary looks after him.

When a mother feels overwhelmed by the child I show or tell her a soothing tale which is partly congruent with the feelings of persecution the child can engender. It can relieve the tension, move from the personal to the general, and help to look at the family situation in a reflective way.

The Cuckoo: A Siberian Tale

There was once a woman with four children who would never obey her. From dawn to dusk they tumbled and rolled in the snow until, at the end of the day, their clothes were wet and torn.

Of course their poor mother had to dry and mend them. And when they trod snow in the tent she had to sweep it out. The mother did the fishing, the cooking, the cleaning and the curing of skins with no help from anyone. Her life was full of suffering and one day she fell ill.

As she lay in her bed she called to her children, 'My children obey your mother this once I beg of you. My throat is so dry; bring me water from the stream.'

The unhappy woman waited in her bed. But no one answered her call.

It was not until evening that her children, hungry and tired, entered the tent and were surprised to find their mother struggling to put on her old grey cloak. How astonished they were to see the cloak suddenly become covered in grey feathers. And then as she reached up to take her hide-curing board, it turned into a bird's tail. Her leather thimble became a beak and her arms turned into wings. The poor woman had turned into a bird.

'Look, look, mother is flying away,' shouted the eldest child, as the bird flew out of the tent and up into the blue sky.

The four children rushed after her crying: 'Mother, mother, come back, we'll bring you water.'

But on the wind came back a call. 'Cuc-koo, cuc-koo, cuc-koo. Too late, too late, too late.'

For two full moons the children ran after their mother, stumbling over rocks and tufts of grass, following the curves of land that led across the tundra. Soon their bare feet were torn and bleeding so that they left a crimson trail wherever they ran. But the mother had abandoned her family for good.

Since that time, the cuckoo has never built a nest, nor raised her own children. And red moss is sprinkled like red drops of blood across the barren tundra.

Helping adults and children connect together

For children with attachment disorders we need to offer simple nurture in moments of relaxation, but in a way which does not overwhelm or threaten. Many children fear physical contact and that should be respected until the child comes to you. Other children are too free with physical contact and it is up to the adults to direct the child to the carers as nurturers. When these children are adopted it is often difficult for the parents to inform friends and relatives that this over-friendly little person is displaying a lack of attachment.

Some of these issues are also present in children who, for whatever reason, have limited understanding of the meaning of social interaction. Here are some ways for carers to develop attachment or help soothe children who are anxious about the meaning of connection to other people.

Music

Try the following:

- Listen to music together.

- Talk about favourite artists; listen to fast/slow tunes.

- Try dancing/rapping together to favourite songs.

- Connect favourite songs to memories of people and/or places.

Rhymes and songs

With young children use playful rhymes and lullabies you can sing or play together. The rhythm of the rhymes and repetition of the lines and phrases create soothing patterns and help attunement between carer and child. While the rhymes may seem simple the structure and rhythm create a safe boundary between adult and child. As the child connects with the rhymes, he or she might be more able to accept nurture in play. If you were lucky enough to have parents who played with you then those happy memories will pass on from you to the child. I still remember saying the following rhyme with my father when I was very small, in the house and in the air raid shelter during the Second World War, and in

times of stress as an adult the comfort of the rhyme and memories of my
father still soothe me.

Two Little Grey Birds

Two little grey birds sat on a stone,
One flew away, and then there was one;
T'other flew after, and then there was none;
So the poor stone was left all alone.
One of the grey birds back again flew,
T'other came after, and then there were two;
Said one to t'other – How do you do?
Very well Ann, and how are you?

For the child who is learning to make jokes:

I Went Up One Pair of Stairs

A: I went up one pair of stairs,
B: Just like me.
A: I went up two pairs of stairs,
B: Just like me.

A: I went into a room,
B: Just like me.
A: I looked out of a window,
B: Just like me.
A: And there I saw a monkey,
B: Just like me!

A Canner

A canner exceedingly canny
One morning remarked to his granny
'A canner can can
Anything that he can
But a canner can't can a can, can he?'

'Cheer up' rhymes:

One, Two, Whatever You Do

One, two, whatever you do,
Start it well and carry it through.
Try, try, never say die,
Things will come right, you know, by-and-by.

Little Jumping Joan

Here I am little jumping Joan,
When nobody's with me
I'm always alone.

With Flowers on My Shoulders

With flowers on my shoulders
And slippers on my feet
I'm my mother's darling
Don't you think I'm sweet?

For the chaotic child, some laughter and the thought that it happens to others too:

Diddle Diddle Dumpling

Diddle diddle dumpling, my son, John,
Went to bed with his trousers on;
One shoe off, the other shoe on,
Diddle diddle dumpling, my son, John.

And other children can also fall out over nothing:

Coffee and Tea

Milly, my sister, and I fell out,
And what do you think it was all about?
She loved coffee, and I loved tea,
And that was the reason we couldn't agree.

And just to be soothed:

A Walnut

There was a little green house,
And in the little green house,
There was a little brown house,
And in the little brown house,
There was a little yellow house,
And in the little yellow house,
There was a little white house,
And in the little white house,
There was a little heart.

Smiling Girls, Rosy Boys

Smiling girls and rosy boys,
Come and buy my little toys,
Monkeys made of gingerbread,
And sugar horses painted red.

Role-playing

Children who do not understand the meaning of social interaction are often 'talked at' by adults or are given long verbal explanations about why their behaviour with others is not considered acceptable. Playing a scene then looking at different ways of responding can be a more helpful way to explore social interaction. But start with simple interactions before starting role-play. Here are some suggestions:

- *Balloons.* Child and adult try to blow up a balloon. Good for breathing. Adult and child each have a balloon and must keep the balloon in the air by blowing or patting with the hand. Play both sitting and standing.

- *Pass the mask.* Adult makes a funny face, child copies the face, passes the expression back to the adult who wipes the expression away by stroking the face with the hand, then makes another expression to pass back to the child.

- *Water cup game.* Have a plastic beaker full of water. Pass from adult to child and back without spilling.

- *Things we do together.* Mime things to do together. For example, folding a sheet, fastening a necklace. Develop with talking as you complete the task.

- *Pass the hat.* Have a selection of hats. Begin just passing a hat from adult to child. With older children develop a character who might wear the hat. Choose a hat each, invent a character for the hat, have a conversation in character with each other.

- *Park bench.* The scene is a park bench on a sunny afternoon. Adult and child choose a hat and decide on a character. They meet on the park bench and start a conversation. Try to make friends with each other.

CHANGING THE STATEMENT

Elaborate on the statements and make a little drama scene.

> A: My teacher always yells at us.
> B: Always? She would explode.

> A: I will always be last to be picked for the football team.
> B: Always?

To end play

After playing together always end with a soothing activity. Try relaxing in a chair, listen to a favourite piece of music, or a good long stretch with a sigh. Then perhaps a story.

Snow White in the Forest (Russian)

Once upon a time there lived an old man and an old woman. They had a little granddaughter called Snow White. Snow White's playmates made up a party once to go to the forest for berries and they came to ask Snow White to go with them. For a long time the old people would not let Snow White go but at last they agreed, telling her that she must not wander away from her friends.

The little girls came to the forest and began to collect berries. Snow White soon wandered away from her friends. They called to her but Snow White did not hear them. Soon it began to grow dark and the little girls went home. Snow White went on and on through the forest until she was quite lost. When she knew that she was all alone in the forest she climbed up a tree and sat on a branch. She began to cry:

> Granddad and granny had a darling little girl,
> Hear her cry and moan.
> Her playmates took her to the woods
> And left her all alone.

A bear came along and said: 'What are you crying for, Snow White?'

'Haven't I good cause to cry, Mr Bear? I'm Snow White and the only grandchild of my granddad and granny. My playmates took me to the woods and left me all alone.'

'Climb down from the tree and I'll take you home to your granddad and granny,' said the bear.

'No, I'm afraid you'll eat me.'

The bear went away and left her.

She began to cry again and to sing her song.

> Poor little Snow White,
> Hear her cry and moan.
> Her playmates took her to the woods
> And left her all alone.

A wolf came along and said, 'What are you crying for, Snow White?'

She answered him just as she had answered the bear.

'Come down,' said the wolf, 'and I'll carry you home to your granddad and granny.'

'No, I'm afraid of you. You'll eat me.'

The wolf went away and Snow White began to cry again and sing her song. Mrs Fox came running by. She heard Snow White's little voice and she said: 'What are you crying for, Snow White?'

'Haven't I good cause to cry, Mrs Fox? My playmates took me to the woods and left me all alone.'

'Come down and I'll carry you to your granddad and granny.'

Snow White climbed down from the tree and jumped onto the fox's back. Off they went at a trot. The fox soon reached Snow White's home and knocked on the door with her tail.

'Who's there?' said the granddad and granny.

'It's Mrs Fox. I've brought your little granddaughter home.'

'Ah, is that our little darling? Come into the cottage, Mrs Fox, sit down and have something to eat.'

They brought milk and eggs and served the fox with a grand feast. Mrs Fox asked if they would give her a hen for a reward. The old folk gave her a white hen, and then they let her go into the forest.

It takes a very long time to establish trust between carers and children who find social interaction confusing. It can be dispiriting and sometimes the adults feel they are drowning, deskilled and unloved. So the basis of nurturing others is firstly to nurture yourself.

A story for the adults

Sometimes at the end of a hard day, when children have rejected us and we wonder why we do what we do, it is good to nurture ourselves with chocolate and a good story. I enjoy this somewhat strange Inuit story about the getting of children, describing the struggle and the desire. This yearning for children is often forgotten after a hard day with a child who is afraid to make any warm connection. The reverse world described in the story, where babies are bigger than adults, reminds me of the way children who struggle with attachment try to control the family.

Kakuarshuk

Long ago women got their children by digging around in the earth. They would pry the children from the ground. Girls were easy to find, for boys you had to travel further. They were more difficult to locate and you would have to dig very deep to find a boy.

Strong women had many children because they could dig deep. But gentlewomen had few children and there were barren women as well. Kakuarshuk was one of the barren women. She would spend nearly all her time digging up the ground. She seemed to turn over half the earth but she found no children. At last she went to a wise woman who told her to go to a place far away and she would find a child. Kakuarshuk went to that place so far away and she began to dig. Deeper and deeper she dug until she came to the other side of the earth. On this side everything seemed to be in reverse. There was no snow and ice and babies were much bigger than adults.

Kakuarshuk was adopted by two of these babies, a girl baby and a boy baby; they carried her around and gave her food and attention.

One day her baby mother said, 'Is there anything you want, Dear Little One?'

'Yes,' Kakuarshuk replied, 'I would like to have a baby of my own.'

'In that case,' her baby mother replied, 'you must go far up in the mountains and there you must start digging.'

And so Kakuarshuk travelled deep into the mountains. She dug and dug. Deeper and deeper the hole went until it joined many other holes. None of these holes appeared to have an exit anywhere. Nor did Kakuarshuk find any babies along the way. But still she walked on. At night she was visited by Claw-Trolls who tore at her flesh. At last she could walk no further and she lay down to die. Suddenly a little fox came up to her, 'I will save you mother, just follow me,' and the fox took her by the hand and led her through the network of holes until they found daylight on the other side.

Kakuarshuk could not remember a thing, not a thing. But when she woke she was resting in her own house and there was a little boy child in her arms.

CHAPTER 5

School

Learn willingly, dear grandson, do not curse the control of the grim teacher. Never shudder at the teacher's appearance. His age may make him frightening, and his harsh words and frowning brows may lead you to think that he wants to pick a quarrel with you – but once you've trained your face to remain impassive, he will never again seem an ogre.

Ausonius, professor of grammar and rhetoric, to his six-year-old grandson, fourth century CE (Wiedemann 1989)

My dear, dear Mother,
If you don't let me come home, I die – I am all over ink, and my fine clothes have been spoilt – I have been tost in a blanket, and seen a ghost.
I remain, my dear, dear mother
Your most dutiful and most
Unhappy son,
Freddy

PS Remember me to my father.

Letter from Frederick Reynolds, aged about seven, after two days at Westminster School, London, 1750

School as chaos

Through the ages it would seem that for some children school is a frightening and miserable place, with teachers who are scary and other children who tease and torment you. Children who find social relationships confusing and don't understand the reasons for rules can struggle to find a meaning for school. Amy, aged 12, had been told that she was stupid from a very early age. She worried about school because she thought she wouldn't understand the teacher. Here is her story once again:

The Person with Very Little Brain

This person could be anyone.
They were born with very little brain and need to get sorted.
Somebody was making fun saying:
'You don't have a very good brain.'

Although Amy had caring adoptive parents she still found school a struggle because she was afraid she couldn't learn. She had also moved to a new school at the age of 11, the other children already knew each other, so she was the odd one out. However, with the support of loving adoptive parents and a sympathetic teacher she has found a place for herself in the class. Her teacher gave the class a positive narrative about the 'new girl' so that her classmates wanted to show her around and tell her the dos and don'ts of her new school. Amy settled well, learnt to make friends and realized very quickly that she had a very large brain and could learn if she kept calm and concentrated. Her mother and the teacher helped her to curb her desire to parent everyone and both adults gave her explanations about school rules and why they were necessary. It is so important for parent and teacher to work together to support the child so the teacher has an understanding of the reasons for the child's behaviour.

Amy's brother Terry, aged eight, had a different struggle. He found it very difficult to concentrate and to curb his swearing. He was able to make friends with other children but he was constantly afraid that he would swear and get into trouble. Like many children who have experienced abuse he was also afraid to use the school lavatory so had to rush home at lunchtime and after school to relieve himself. Again teachers understood, developing strategies to help Terry. A classroom support worker took him to the playground for a five-minute stretch and body shake after each lesson to help him relax and concentrate. I was helping him settle with his new family and he was allowed at the beginning of each session with me to swear if he needed and get rid of the tension on the understanding that he controlled that urge when he was in school or in the playground. Terry enjoyed his sessions with me, and initially he spewed out his swear words non-stop for five minutes. My response was one of indifference and later boredom with his language. Over the weeks he also became indifferent to bad language, as it had no shock value between us, so it stopped. He was also able to control his language in school. He had lapses at home but gradually learnt that his language didn't arouse adults in the way he wanted and only got him in trouble, which might mean less time with his mini motor bike.

As the children settled in home and school their attachment patterns shifted and they began to trust their new parents and their schoolteachers. Their social environment, living in a small village, helped to secure their sense of belonging. There were still developmental issues left over from early abuse and neglect. Any changes to their routine brought anxiety and inappropriate responses. When they are anxious they test the boundaries just to make sure about the rules and to check whether the adults will reject them. They are at times over-familiar with acquaintances and spill out family information to all, but they feel accepted as part of a family and a community.

Rules

One of the difficulties experienced by children who are confused by social interaction is to understand the way the school day is structured and what rules of behaviour mean in a school setting. Simon is preparing to go to senior school. He has found primary school difficult, struggling to keep control of his behaviour in the classroom. He is getting help from the educational psychologist to prepare him for the school move. Simon finds change very upsetting so his parents are to visit the senior school with him and speak to his teacher about how the school day is organized. He will be able to make several visits with his parents to familiarize himself with the school and how to move around the building. Simon is pleased and excited about these visits because he says he was very worried about how he would manage. Simon knows that he forgets the rules of the classroom when the noise level rises and he loses concentration.

I read to Simon from *The School of Manners* (1983), written in 1701, about what was expected of 'Behaviour in the School'. He enjoyed thinking about those boys of long ago and what was expected of them.

We could talk about the rules together, comparing and contrasting the past with what was expected today. He didn't feel nagged or blamed when we looked at these rules and he felt free to talk about his school and reflect about rules and what and who they were there to help. Some of the rules in 1701 were very sensible, others a bit strict for modern times. We both liked the idea of a very flashy school hat, which could be removed with a dramatic gesture coming into school. Children who are impulsive find it difficult to reflect on their own behaviour through confrontational discourse but can be reflective using imaginative processes.

Of Behaviour in the School (1701)

1. Bow coming in, Putting off thine hat; especially if the Master or Other is present.

2. Loiter not but immediately take thine own seat, and move not from one place to another till School time be over.

3. If any stranger come into the School, rise up and bow, and sit down in thy place again, keeping a profound silence.

4. If the Master be discoursing in the School with a stranger, stare not confidently on them, nor hearken to their talk.

5. Interrupt not the Master while a stranger or a visitor is with him, with any question, request or complaint; but defer any such matter till he be at leisure.

6. At no time talk or quarrel in the School; but be quiet peaceable and silent: Much less mayest thou deceive thyself by trifling away the time in play.

7. If thy Master speak to thee, rise up and bow, making thine answer standing.

8. Bawl not aloud in making complaints: A Boys tongue should be never heard in school but in answering a question or repeating his lesson.

9. If a stranger speak to thee in school stand up and answer with respect and ceremony, both of words and gesture, as if thou speakest to thy Master.

10. Make not haste out of school, but soberly go when thy turn comes, without notice or hurry.

11. Go not rudely home through the street, stand not talking with boys to delay thee, but go quietly home, and with all convenient haste.

12. Divulge not to any person whatever elsewhere, any thing that hath passed in the School either spoken or done.

School as sanctuary

Some children who struggle to find a place in family life find school a safe place to be and learn. Perhaps because nobody wants to parent them and affection isn't demanded they can relax. However, although adults, especially teachers, respond to children who want to learn sometimes there are difficulties with other children. This is Mary's story:

> There was once a black girl called No Name.
> And she was nice.
> She liked her hair like that, it made her feel a feeling,
> But she didn't want to tell.
> She wore short socks and shoes
> But the shoes smelt sweaty
> And this made her feel different from all the other children.
> Because she was different
> She decided to be better than everybody else.
> She was good at absolutely everything,
> Maths, Music, Reading, Running, Singing, Acting.
> She was not so good at English, History, PE, RE, French.
> She came top of the class in all the things she was good at.
> No Name's best friend is a girl called No Voice
> Who doesn't speak because she is sad.
> If she spoke, her story would be so terribly sad
> That she would be afraid.
> So No Voice has no voice.
> She is good at school too.

For the teachers, Mary was a delight to teach and no trouble in class. The classroom was Mary's haven and she felt safe there, wanted, respected and admired by adults for her learning skills. However, she did struggle to make friends with the other children but because she was so well behaved in class her problems were not considered to be important. Gradually the lack of friends worried Mary and she became reluctant to go to school. She eventually made one good friend and together they were able to cope with their classmates and maintain the respect of their teachers.

Alice was 14 and she too was well behaved in class and gained excellent marks in all her school subjects. All the teachers liked her and she was easy to teach. She found the learning process in school enhanced her self-esteem and she felt safe when she was working. Her difficulties, as for Mary, lay in making appropriate friendships. When she was living with her birth family Alice parented her two siblings and she used this model of communication with her peers. They resented her desire to control their behaviour so there were many splits in friendships. Alice also felt obliged to mediate rows between groups in school as she saw her role as to make everyone happy. The other girls resented this and some girls began to bully Alice who then became reluctant to go to school.

Alice also suffered flashbacks about the physical abuse she experienced as a young child. If the noise in school became too intense, Alice became very anxious and lost concentration. Because Alice was quiet and polite in the classroom, initially her fears were dismissed and nothing was done to support her. Her adoptive mother tried many times to explain Alice's needs to staff but again this was dismissed. It was only after intervention by the educational psychologist that Alice's needs were recognized and she was able to go and sit in the school nurse's office when she felt fearful. Alice and I worked out strategies to help her relax after school and to analyse Alice's interactions with her friends. We shifted some of the inappropriate mothering approaches and helped Alice recognize that she wasn't responsible for the happiness of her school class. Alice felt that when she came to live with her adoptive family she was worthless and that it had taken six years' learning how to behave for her to become loveable. We discussed this view of herself and it was challenged by all her family who told her that she was always loveable and didn't have to be made so by her family. Alice wrote about her school experiences:

Bad Experience

In my secondary school there are good experiences and bad experiences. One of my bad experiences in school which ended quite recently was in drama. I'm not really a confident person so I don't always do well in this subject but to make matters worse there was this girl in my class who was really nasty to me and made going to drama really hard.

Eventually I stopped going to class and my guidance teacher was informed. I spoke to my mum about it and she battled with my guidance teacher for weeks, but the situation didn't get any better. My guidance teacher wasn't willing to do anything about it because there wasn't a witness to anything. I didn't have anyone in the class to back me and the teacher never saw anything. I felt really upset and lonely because I felt like I had no friend in the class.

As I gained in confidence I started going to class again. And I learnt to ignore the girl who was horrible to me. It wasn't easy but I got through it in one piece.

Good Experience

One of the good experiences was when I was in PE because it is my best subject and I really feel like I can achieve something from it. I have never missed a PE lesson and I always bring my kit.

All the PE staff are really nice and my teacher, who is the Head of Department, has given me great encouragement and is really nice and supportive and I really feel like I can trust her. Recently I received a certificate in the post in recognition of my achievements in PE.

I think I will do really well in this subject and like I said my teacher has given me great encouragement and is really pleased that I am taking PE at a Standard Grade.

I have more kind teachers than unkind and I feel safe and supported in most of my classes and I hope to carry on doing well in school and go on to pass all my exams.

Strategies for teachers helping children with attachment difficulties

Children and young people with attachment difficulties have inappropriate social relatedness with their peers and adults. This can take the form of inhibited or disinhibited responses to most social interactions. There are a variety of strategies the teacher can employ in order to keep such pupils safe in school.

- Be predictable, consistent and repetitive to alleviate fear of change. Students become anxious about changes in timetables, surprises and chaotic social situations.

- Model and teach appropriate social behaviours. Role-play for the student, then narrate what is happening, then ask the student to role-play.

- Avoid power struggles. Students with attachment issues usually want to be in control and if they receive an emotional response they will feel they have hooked you into their world and have won a power battle.

- Break down information into manageable segments for the purposes of comprehension. This can alleviate anxiety and the desire to give up on learning.

- Find a place for the student to go to regain composure during times of frustration or fear, for example the nurse's room at school.

Bullying

Nerd's Story

There was once a Nerd that went to a shop
And in that shop people didn't like Nerds.
They were all drinking in the shop.
The Nerd wanted some crisps and the shopman said,
'Nerds aren't allowed to buy anything here.
If you do it's £3 extra.'
The Nerd got angry.
'Who do you think you are talking to?
I earn more than you.
You are just a drunkard.'
Then the drunkard got really angry
And he took out both of the Nerd's eyes.
He put them in the Nerd's mouth
And made him swallow them.
The Nerd nearly died.
He was just lucky enough to live.
The Nerd grew two more eyes.

This was Jamie's pretend story about being bullied. He was eight years old and was teased at school because he was 'different'. His classmates knew he was in care and thought it was legitimate to bully him. Jamie felt really bad about himself, he thought he was a Nerd and his classmates sensed his vulnerability. Jamie didn't have the words to answer back and knew that when he got angry he could lash out at his classmates and then he would be in trouble with the teacher. The bullying at school reminded him of the violence he had experienced from his father when he lived at home. He felt his choice was to endure the bullies or become a bully himself.

Peer group rejection

The research on peer group rejection by Newcomb and Bukowski (1984) indicates that some rejected children are immature, others socially unskilled, others rejected because of their aggressive behaviour and still yet others because they are socially wary and withdrawn. Newcomb, Bukowski and Pattee (1993) found that rejected children lack positive social actions, positive social traits and friendships. Dodge (1983) considers that their methods for initiating group entry differ greatly from those popular children and may explain their continual rejection. For example, rejected children tend to hover and wait for invitations to join a peer group and then rapidly switch to high-risk tactics that disrupt the group.

Definitions of bullying

There are many definitions of bullying. Kidscape information on the Internet defines physical bullying, verbal bullying and emotional bullying, which includes being tormented, ridiculed and humiliated. ChildLine information on the Internet lists the following types of bullying that have been the concerns of children and young people who have called their helpline:

- being teased or called names
- being hit, pushed, pulled, pinched or kicked
- having their bags, mobiles, money or other possessions taken

- receiving abusive text messages or emails

- being ignored or left out

- being attacked or abused because of religion, gender, sexuality, disability, appearance or ethnic or racial origin.

ChildLine (2007) has good advice for children and young people who are being bullied:

ChildLine's top tips

1. Don't ignore bullying, it won't go away on it's own and it may get worse.

2. Tell someone you trust – such as a teacher, parent or friend.

3. Remember it's not your fault. No one deserves to be bullied.

Here are some other things you might want to think about:

1. Keep a record – and save any nasty texts or emails that you have been sent.

2. Try to stay away from the bullies or stay with a group when you don't feel safe.

3. Ask your mates to look out for you.

4. Try not to retaliate – you could get into trouble or get hurt.

5. Check your school's anti-bullying policy. This will tell you what your school should do about bullying.

6. Try to act more confident – even if you don't feel it.

7. Call ChildLine for extra help on 0800 1111.

There is also advice for children who bully:

- You do have a choice – just because you've bullied others in the past doesn't mean you have to keep doing it.

- People who are bullied can feel upset and scared. You can put a stop to that by changing your behaviour.

- Sometimes things happen to you that make you more likely to bully others – being bullied yourself, for instance, or having problems at home. It's important to get help for yourself, rather than take your frustrations out on others.

Jamie worked on his communication skills and we did a lot of role-play together changing his presentation of self so his physical stance and walk indicated a more confident person. Ignoring and not listening to taunts was the best way for Jamie to cope with bullying. Verbal responses were difficult for him. We used an image of Dr Who in his Tardis, which he thought about as he walked through the group who were abusive to him. He felt secure imagining himself safe in the Tardis, so managed to ignore the insults of the group. Jamie felt powerful as he learnt to cope and his desire to bully others left him. He knew what it felt like and didn't want to instil that fear into others. It was still a temptation to fight back with his fists when someone made a nasty remark but Jamie managed to control himself most of the time. He didn't want to be excluded from school. Jamie recognized that while some bullies appeared to be popular with classmates it was partly through fear. He didn't want to be feared, he wanted to be a winner and make some friends, and he knew he must try to manage his behaviour to achieve the place in his class which he wanted. We used role-play to explore ways to enter a group and the verbal and non-verbal skills required to gain acceptance. We repeated these scenes many times until Jamie could respond automatically. Then we developed more complicated role-play.

Role-play examples

IDENTIFICATION AND EMPATHY

This involves two players. Player one makes a true statement; for example, 'It's snowing today.'

Player two has to interpret what player one has said by asking, 'Do you mean…?' Player one answers yes or no to the question depending on how accurate the question seems to be.

Continue asking questions until player one answers yes three times. For example:

Player 1: 'It's snowing today.'

Player 2: 'Do you mean you like to see snow?'

Player 1: 'Yes.'

Player 2: 'Do you mean you are cold?'

Player 1: 'No.'

Player 2: 'Do you mean you can't get to school?'

Player 1: 'Yes.'

...and so on.

CONFLICTING ROLES

Make a short scene with two players: one player the teacher, the other the student.

Start with this dialogue:

Teacher: 'Pay attention please.'

Student: 'You're picking on me.'

Play the scene for three minutes, improvising dialogue. Players then reverse role and play the scene again. Discuss what it felt like playing both roles.

NEW AT SCHOOL

New student meets classmate. Dialogue begins with new student: 'Excuse me, I'm new here.' Improvise a scene with dialogue for three minutes. Then reverse roles and improvise the scene again. Which role did you like best and why?

Support from carers

No child or young person should be bullied and all bullying should be reported. It is sometimes difficult for carers to know if their child is being bullied because many children fear the responses of parents, thinking it will make matters worse. They don't want to upset their parents, or they feel their parents won't take them seriously or will just tell them to stand up for themselves.

Carers need to spend time with their child to ask about school and check what is happening there. If you observe changes in behaviour like anger, nervousness, poor sleep or nightmares, then gently ask the child to explain. If the child says they are being bullied it is important to listen and let the child tell their story in their own words. If the child won't talk about it suggest that they talk to another adult who they trust.

Once it is established that a child is being bullied it is important for carers not to rush in demanding to meet the bully's family or to blame the head or the teacher. This is what children dread the most and makes them afraid to talk with their carers.

Suggest that the child keep a diary of all the incidents and make an appointment to meet with the teacher together. If the bullying persists keep on reporting it to the school.

Kidscape (2007) lists the top ten frustrations of parents of bullied children as follows:

1. No response to letters or phone calls.

2. Being told a child is: fussing, over-sensitive, needs to 'laugh it off'.

3. Promising verbally to do things which don't happen.

4. No blame approach.

5. Asking repeatedly for school's anti-bullying policy.

6. Being told that the bullying 'has been dealt with internally' and given no details.

7. No consequences for the bullies – 'they've been spoken to'.

8. Their children having to move classes or offered lunch in the library, a counsellor etc., while the bully goes free.

9. Family rows/upsets/divorce because of bullying.

10. Being told 'we don't have bullying in this school'.

The *Kidscape* website also gives advice on how to deal with these frustrations: www.kidscape.org.uk. There are sensible suggestions to combat these frustrations. Carers become very anxious and feel powerless when they want to support the child and stop the bullying but might have to fight many levels of bureaucracy to be heard. Check the school's anti-bullying policy. There is a legal responsibility for all schools to have a written anti-bullying policy and you can check that the policy is being implemented.

Schools

There are many ways for schools to implement their bullying policy and not have parents experience the ten frustrations described above. First find out the extent of bullying in the school, perhaps using questionnaires or discussions at parents' evenings. Then there should be a clear structure in place for all staff to know how to deal with each incident of bullying. All the staff need to deal with incidents in the same way using the school structures. There is nothing more frustrating for the carers and child if there are no clear procedures.

Bullying prevention programmes

There have been a variety of bullying prevention programmes; the Olweus Prevention Programme (Olweus and Limber 1998) launched in Norway and Sweden in the 1980s is one example. This is a multilevel, multicomponent school-based programme designed to reduce or prevent bullying in pupils aged 6–15. Core programme components are implemented at the school, classroom and individual levels.

School-wide components include:

- the administration of an anonymous questionnaire to assess the nature and prevalence of bullying at each school
- training for all staff
- formation of bullying prevention coordinating committee
- increased supervision at 'hotspots' for bullying
- development of school-wide rules against bullying
- consistent consequences for following/not following the rules
- a school-wide kick-off event
- parental involvement
- staff discussion groups to ensure understanding and motivation.

Classroom components include:

- holding regular classroom meetings with pupils about bullying

- consistent reinforcement of school rules against bullying.

Individual components include:

- interventions with children identified as bullies and victims
- discussions with parents of involved children.

Massage routines

Anti-bullying programmes address issues mainly through cognitive approaches, and the introduction of massage programmes in schools can perhaps help develop nurturing touch in a school setting. These Massage in Schools Programmes are based on respect for the other person and involves a formal massage routine. The clothed peer massage is for children 4–12 years old, given and received with the child's permission, given by the children to each other, on the back, head, arms and hands for 10–15 minutes daily. Trained instructors teach the children the daily massage routine. One of the results of these programmes is a reduction in bullying and aggressive behaviour in the school.

Peer support in school

One of the most helpful ways to support children having difficulties with bullying and making friends is with peer support. Finding a caring older person who understands the school because he/she is also a student can be very helpful.

Cowie (2004) states that peer support offers a system of assistance where young people's potential to be helpful can be fostered through appropriate training and through the support of regular debriefing sessions. These systems include befriending schemes, where peer supporters are trained to offer friendship or support in everyday interaction with peers, and mentoring schemes where the peer supporter, usually an older pupil, is trained to offer positive role modelling through a one-to-one relationship with a younger or vulnerable peer.

Johnny, aged 14, has Asperger's syndrome and is being bullied in school. He now has a mentor, an older student, and they meet on a regular basis. Andrew, his mentor, supports Johnny in a variety of ways. They play football together, which helps Johnny's co-ordination, and they role-play communication situations when Johnny might be bullied. Johnny now has a strategy to switch off from the verbal disrespect by imagining he is a racing driver in his car, and so not vulnerable to taunts as he drives through the crowd. Both young men enjoy their time together, so it is a learning experience for both Johnny and Andrew in making good relationships.

Johnny likes the story *A Pottle o' Brains* because the message that there is always someone who likes you the way you are is full of hope for him.

A Pottle o' Brains

Once in these parts, and not so long ago, there was a boy who wanted to buy a pottle o' brains, for he was always getting into scrapes because of his foolishness, and being laughed at by everyone.

Folk told him he could get everything he liked from the wise woman that lived on the top of the hill, and dealt in potions and herbs and spells and things. She could even tell the future.

So the boy asked his mother if he could seek the old woman and buy a pottle o' brains.

'Yes you can,' said his mother. 'You are in great need of them, and if I die who would take care of such a fool as you who has no more idea of looking after yourself than a newborn baby? But mind your manners when you speak to her because such wise folk are quickly displeased.'

So off he went, after his tea, and there she was, sitting by the fire, stirring a big pot.

'Good evening, missis,' he says, 'it's a fine night.'

'Aye,' says she and went on stirring.

'It'll maybe rain,' says he and fidgets from one foot to the other.

'Maybe,' says she.

'And happen it won't,' says he and looks out of the window.

'Happen,' says she.

And he scratched his head and twisted his cap. 'Well,' says he, 'I can't mind nothing else about the weather, but let me see, the crops are getting on fine.'

'Fine,' says she. 'And-the-beasts-is-fattening,' says he.

'They are,' says she.

'And, and, and,' then he comes to a stop. 'I reckon we'll tackle business now having done the polite like. Have you any brains to sell?'

'That depends,' says she. 'If you want a king's brains, or a soldier's brains or a schoolmaster's brains, I dinna keep them.'

'Oh no,' says he, 'just ordinary brains, same as everyone has around here, something clean, common like.'

'Aye so,' says the old woman.' 'I might manage that if you'll help yourself.'

'How do I do that missis?' says he.

'Bring me the heart of the thing you like best of all, and I'll tell you where to get your pottle o' brains, but you'll have to read me a riddle, so as I can see you've brought the right thing, and if your brain is about you.'

'But,' says he, scratching his head, 'how can I do that?'

'That's not for me to say. Find out for yourself my lad.'

So the boy went back home and told his mother what had happened.

'I reckon I'll have to kill the pig,' says he, 'for I like fat bacon better than anything.'

So he killed the pig and next day set off for the old woman's cottage.

'Good-day,' he said. 'I've brought you the heart of the thing I love best.'

'Aye so,' said she and looked at him through her spectacles. 'Tell me this then, what runs without feet?'

He scratched his head and thought and thought but couldn't tell.

'Go thy ways,' said the old woman. 'You haven't fetched me the right thing yet.'

So off the boy went to tell his mother but as he got to his house, out came folk running to tell him his mother was dying. When he got in, his mother smiled because she thought he had his brains and then she died.

The boy was very sad because he remembered how kind his mother had been to him and how she had looked after him so well and put up with his foolishness. Then he realized that his mother was the one he loved the best but he couldn't cut out her heart to bring to the old woman. So he put his mother into a sack and carried her body to the old woman's cottage.

'Good-day missis,' says he. 'I think I've fetched the right thing this time.'

'Maybe,' said the old woman, 'but read me this, now what's yellow and shining but isn't gold?'

He scratched his head, and thought, but couldn't tell.

'Thou hast not hit the right thing yet,' said the old woman. 'You are more foolish than I thought.'

The boy left and sat down by the roadside.

'I've lost the only two things I care for. What else can I find to buy a pottle o' brains?' And he began to cry.

And up came a girl who lived nearby and asked him what had happened and he told her about the old woman and the pottle o' brains and that he was now alone in the world.

'Well I wouldn't mind looking after you,' said the girl. 'People like you make good husbands.'

They got married and decided to wait a bit before going to see the old woman again.

The boy and girl were very happy together and, after a while, the boy told the girl that she was now the person he liked best of everything. 'But I'm not going to cut out your heart for a pottle o' brains.'

'I'm glad to hear it,' said the girl. 'You take me to see the old woman and I'll help you read the riddles.'

'I reckon they are too hard for womenfolk,' said he.

'Well let's see now. Tell me the first.'

'What runs without feet?'

'Why, water,' says she.

'And what is yellow and shining and not gold?'

'Why, the sun,' says she.

'That's right,' says he. 'Come, we'll go to the old woman.'

So off they went.

The old woman was sitting outside twining straws.

'Good-day missis,' says he. 'I reckon I've fetched the right thing at last.'

The wise woman looked at them both.

'Canst tell me what that is as has first no legs, and then two legs, and ends with four legs?'

And the boy scratched his head but couldn't tell. And the girl whispered in his ear: 'It's a tadpole.'

The boy told the old woman, who nodded her head.

'That's right, and you have your pottle o' brains already.'

'Where be they?' he asked searching in his pockets.

'In your wife's head,' says she.

So they went home together and he never wanted to buy a pottle o' brains again, for his wife had enough for both.

Friendship

This is Pamela's story about friendship. She has mild learning difficulties. She enjoys school and is popular with her classmates and younger children. She was 14 when she wrote this story. As Pamela tells the story she sometimes switches from third-person narration to first-person narration then back again. The description of playing with a friend is what excites Pamela and sucks her into her own story. She loves to play with a friend and in her reality world she has learnt to negotiate with others as they play and work together.

The Island of Happiness

This is a nice island. It is cool.
Not too warm and not too cold.
Pamela the dinosaur lives there
With her furry friend who is a smaller dinosaur.
They climb trees and at the top they jump down squealing.
One day two aliens come to the island.
They were very nasty.
They tried to take Pamela's furry friend
But Pamela bit them and they ran away.
And we were climbing on other trees,
A higher one.
We didn't jump, we climbed.
My furry friend went halfway down
Then Pamela jumped.
The parents didn't visit the island
But they would come if Pamela called them.

On the island there are lots of little lakes to swim in.
One day me and the furry creature went swimming
But the furry friend couldn't swim.
So I shared the lake with him and we went swimming together
Instead of climbing trees.
Then he said why didn't we go and do the whole thing again.
The End.

Function of friendship

Rubin *et al.* (2005) suggest that friendships in childhood offer children an extra-familial base of security from which they may explore the effects of their behaviours on themselves, their peers and their environment. As children grow and develop, friendships serve different functions. Parker and Gottman (1989) say that for the young child friendship serves to maximize excitement and amusement levels in play and help organize behaviour in the face of arousal. It would seem that Pamela's description of her friendships describes this function and that is one of the reasons she seeks younger children to befriend because they can play with her in the way she finds fun and helps her feel good about herself.

In middle childhood friendships help in acquiring knowledge about behavioural norms and help children learn the skills necessary for successful self-presentation. These skills become crucial in middle childhood and this is the time when anxiety about peer relationships develops. This is often the time when children who find social under-standing difficult struggle to find and keep friends because they do not always understand how to present themselves in ways which are accept-able to the group.

Sarah is seven and is still trying to find ways to communicate with her peers at school. Her friendships are fragile as she struggles to find ways to communicate. She describes these difficulties in her story:

The Two Crocodiles

Once upon a time there were two crocodiles
And one crocodile had a fish in its mouth.
They played together every day
And some days they had fun
And other days they fought.
When they had fun they sat in the sun

And swam in the river.
When they fought they hit each other very hard
Then went to tell their mothers.
Then they said sorry to each other
But went on fighting.
They stopped fighting when the mothers said,
'Lunch time,' and they both went home to eat.

Laursen, Hartup and Keplas (1996) state that the amount of conflict between friends is greater than between non-friends. Friends resolve these conflicts in ways that help ensure that their relationships persist beyond the conflict and continue in the future. So the crocodiles in Sarah's story stop fighting, go home for food and live to meet and play and fight on another day.

In adolescence friendships serve to assist individuals in their quest for self-exploration and to help them integrate logic and emotions. Many young people who have experienced difficult family relationships struggle with friendships in adolescence. Jane is 14 and finds it difficult to regulate her emotions around her friendships with other young women in her class. Her friendships are 'all or nothing' relationships and can feel overpowering for the recipients. She continually tests the loyalty of her friends and analyses their conversations to check the veracity of their friendship. This can be wearing, so while Jane has friends their relationships are short-lived. Grotpeter and Crick (1996) consider that high levels of relational aggression within the friendship, and high levels of exclusivity, jealousy and intimacy, characterize the friendships of relationally aggressive children. Jane struggled to contain her feelings of jealousy and managed to find a 'best friend' who likes her enough to stay with the stressful times and help her manage her friendships with less intensity.

Rubin et al. (2005) holds that most children have at least one friend. Children become friends with other children who are like themselves in terms of 'surface' characteristics and behavioural characteristics and, during the adolescent years, with others who share similar attitudes, opinions and values. Friends engage in qualitatively different types of interactions than non-friends of all ages, and the characteristics of these interactions can be used to describe and predict the friendship formation process. Although conflict often occurs in friendships, friends resolve conflict in ways that enhance the likelihood that the relationship will persist or continue. Research on children who are without mutual best friends supports the hypothesis that friendship plays a significant role in social development by providing children with settings and contexts within which to learn about themselves, their peers and the world around them.

Encouraging friendships with games

Adults can help children and young people develop social skills which can be transferred to their relationships with their peers:

- Play age-appropriate indoor games with children to help with the winning/losing experience: card games, Connect4, etc.

- Play guessing games around facial expressions. 'Guess what I am feeling by my expression.' Swap roles.

- Play observational games. For example, get all family members together, then choose one person to ask the questions. Questions are around appearance. For example, who is wearing a watch, who has black shoes, etc. Repeat with movement; for example, 'Everyone who is wearing a watch change places.'

- With a larger group make a circle, then the leader calls for everyone who likes ice-cream to stand together, then everyone who likes dogs, cats, Maths lessons, holidays, etc.

This kind of play encourages children to observe others and think of their likes and dislikes.

And, finally, stories can be satisfying. Alice, who at 14 struggles with her friendships, loved the story of *Gobborn Seer* because it describes a clever witty woman who is recognized as such by the family she chooses to marry into.

Gobborn Seer

Gobborn Seer comes from the Irish 'Goban Saor', a travelling carpenter, and a godlike character.

Once there was a man called Gobborn Seer and he had a son called Jack.

One day he sent him out to sell a sheep skin and Gobborn said: 'You must bring me back the skin and the value of it as well.'

So Jack started but he could not find anyone who would leave him the skin and give him its price too. So he came home discouraged.

But Gobborn Seer said, 'Never mind, you must take another turn at it tomorrow.'

So he tried again but nobody wished to buy the sheep skin on those terms. When he came home his father said, 'You must go and try your luck tomorrow,' and the third day it seemed it would be the same thing all over again. And he had half a mind not to go back at all because he thought his father would be angry.

As he came to a bridge he leaned on the parapet thinking of his problem and that it might be foolish to run away from home. But he couldn't tell which to do, when he saw a girl washing her clothes on the bank below.

She looked up and said, 'If it may be no offence asking what is it you feel so badly about.'

'My father has given me this skin and I am to fetch it back and the price of it as well.'

'Is that all? Give it here and it's easily done.'

So the girl washed the skin in the stream, took the wool from it and paid him the value of it, and gave him the skin to carry back. His father was well pleased, and said to Jack, 'That was a witty woman, she would make you a good wife. Do you think you could ask her?'

Jack thought he could, so his father told him to go to the bridge. 'See if she is there and if so ask her to take tea with us.'

And sure enough the girl was there by the bridge and Jack told her that his father would like to meet her and would she like to come home with him and take tea.

The girl thanked him kindly and said she would come the next day as she was very busy at the moment.

'All the better,' said Jack. 'I'll have time to make ready.'

So when she came Gobborn Seer could see she was a witty woman and he asked her if she would marry his Jack.

She said 'Yes' and they were married.

Not long after Jack's father told him he must come with him and build the finest castle that ever was seen for a king who wished to outdo all others by his wonderful castle. And as they went to lay the foundation stone Gobborn Seer said to Jack, 'Can't you shorten the way for me?'

But Jack looked ahead and saw a long road before them and he said, 'I don't see father how I could break a bit off.'

'You're no good to me then and had better be off home.'

So poor Jack turned back and when he came in his wife said, 'Why, how's this you've come alone?'

And he told her what his father had said and his answer.

'You stupid,' said his witty wife. 'If you had told a story you would have shortened the road. Now listen till I tell you a story and then catch up with Gobborn Seer and tell it at once. He will like hearing it and by the time you have done you will have reached the foundation stone.'

So Jack sweated and overtook his father. Gobborn Seer said never a word, but Jack began his story and the road was shortened as his wife had said.

When they came to the end of their journey they started building the castle which was to outshine all others.

Now the wife had advised them to be very friendly with the servants and so they did what she said and said 'Good morning', and 'Good evening', as they passed in and out.

Now at the end of a year Gobborn, the wise man, had built such a castle that thousands were gathered to admire it.

And the king said, 'The castle is done, I shall come tomorrow and pay you all.'

'I have just a ceiling to finish in the upper lobby,' said Gobborn, 'and then it wants nothing.'

But after the king had gone off the housekeeper sent for Gobborn and Jack and told them she had watched for a chance to warn them. For the king was so afraid they would carry their skills away with them and build some other king as fine a castle he meant to take their lives tomorrow.

Gobborn told Jack to keep a good heart and they would come out all right.

When the king came back Gobborn told him he had been unable to complete the job for lack of tools left at home and he should like to send Jack after it.

'No no,' said the king, 'cannot one of the men do the errand?'

'No, they could never make themselves understood,' said the Seer, 'but Jack could do the errand.'

'You and your son are to stop here,' said the king, 'but how if I send my own son?'

'That will do,' said Gobborn Seer.

So Gobborn sent by him a message to Jack's wife, 'Give him crooked and straight.'

Now there was a little hole high up in the wall and Jack's wife tried to reach up into a chest there after crooked and straight. But at last she asked the king's son to help her because his arms were longest.

But when he was leaning over the chest she caught him by the two heels and threw him into the chest and fastened it down. So there he was both 'crooked and straight'.

Then he begged for pen and ink which she brought him but he was not allowed out. And holes were bored so he could breathe.

When the letter came, telling the king, his father, he was to be set free when Gobborn and Jack were safe home, the king saw he must settle for the building and let them come away.

As they left Gobborn told him, now that Jack was done with his work, he should build a castle for his witty wife far superior to the king's.

Which he did, and they lived there happily ever after.

CHAPTER 6

Monsters in My World
Coping with the Adult world

Teeny-Tiny

Once upon a time there was a teeny-tiny woman who lived in a teeny-tiny house in a teeny-tiny village.

Now one day the teeny-tiny woman put on her teeny-tiny bonnet, and went out of her teeny-tiny house to take a teeny-tiny walk.

And when this teeny-tiny woman had gone a teeny-tiny way she came to a teeny-tiny gate, and went into a teeny-tiny churchyard.

And when this teeny-tiny woman had got into the teeny-tiny churchyard, she saw a teeny-tiny bone on a teeny-tiny grave and the teeny-tiny woman said to herself, 'This teeny-tiny bone will make me some teeny-tiny soup for my teeny-tiny supper.'

So the teeny-tiny woman put the teeny-tiny bone into her teeny-tiny pocket and went home to her teeny-tiny house.

Now when the teeny-tiny woman got home to her teeny-tiny house she was a teeny-tiny bit tired so she went up her teeny-tiny stairs to her teeny-tiny bed and put the teeny-tiny bone into a teeny-tiny cupboard.

And when the teeny-tiny woman had been to sleep for some teeny-tiny time she was awakened by a teeny-tiny voice from the teeny-tiny cupboard which said,

'*Give me my bone.*'

And the teeny-tiny woman was a teeny-tiny bit frightened so she hid her teeny-tiny head under the teeny-tiny clothes and went to sleep again.

And when she had been to sleep again for a teeny-tiny time the teeny-tiny voice again cried out from the teeny-tiny cupboard,

'Give me my bone.'

This made the teeny-tiny woman a teeny-tiny more frightened and she hid her teeny-tiny head a teeny-tiny further under the teeny-tiny clothes. And when the teeny-tiny woman had been to sleep again a teeny-tiny time the teeny-tiny voice from the teeny-tiny cupboard said again a teeny-tiny louder,

'Give me my bone.'

And this teeny-tiny woman was a teeny-tiny bit more frightened and she put her teeny-tiny head out of the teeny-tiny clothes, and said in her loudest teeny-tiny voice,

'Take it.'

This story is understood and enjoyed by many of the children with whom I work because, first, it defines what it is like to be physically small and powerless, and second, it describes the fear of a monster in the cupboard. The teeny-tiny woman wisely gives the bone back to the ghost before hiding back in her bed. The story encompasses the experience of being very small, fear of the dark, and of what might lie in the wardrobes, cupboards, under the bed and all the dark places that seem to grow to enormous size in the night. Abused children are often harmed at night, so that feeling of lying scared in bed resonates for many. The repetition of 'teeny-tiny' gives structure and safety to the story and children can join in repeating the words. But most of all it is fun to shout 'give me my bone', and the final 'take it'.

The experience of being physically small and vulnerable in a world of tall strong adults is expressed in many children's narratives. Millie, aged six, in her story describes a baby stuck in slime and although she tries to help the baby in the end the slime and the nasty man are too big and strong and the tiny baby capitulates. So for Teeny Tiny and the tiny baby, surrendering to the monster is their only option. They are too small to offer resistance. Children's struggles in the adult world are the themes of many of their narratives where adults are perceived as monsters.

Millie's Story

There was once a baby who was pushed into the slime
By a naughty man.
She wanted to get out so Millie will take her out.
Some more slime comes along
So Millie will take her out to hide from the slime
Because it is the biggest pile of slime.
The baby gets stuck in the slime.
She cries and says 'No'
But the nasty man says 'Go back in',
He is a big bully.

Warner (1994) in her book and Reith lectures *Managing Monsters* states that children aren't separate from adults, and unlike Mowgli and Peter Pan they can't be kept separate; they can't live innocent lives on behalf of adults. Nor can individuals who happen to be young act as the living embodiment of adults' inner goodness, however much adults may wish it. Without paying attention to adults and their circumstances, children cannot begin to meet the hopes and expectations of our torn dreams about what a child and childhood should be.

Christensen (2000) says that in Denmark the infant is praised for representing that which everyone loses in growing up, that is 'the innocence of childhood'. This view is reflected through children as their increasingly complex nature is perceived to be associated with 'losing' their charm. The child also represents continuity in their similarity to adults and the notion of continuity – that children are expected to survive adults – forms at the same time a challenge to adult control and power.

Children who have experienced difficulties challenge adult expectations about childhood and that can impact on the relationship between the two. Then children lose their individual identity and become those stereotypes 'little devils', 'little angels' rather than intriguing individuals. Children who have been hurt by adults challenge the perceptions of what childhood is supposed to be like. Sometimes the narratives of hurt and abuse overwhelm the adult, who then loses sight of the child behind the story. The adult can only see the child as victim. Then it becomes difficult for the child to confront the adult with their feelings of love and devotion for the perpetrators of hurt. For the adult the child's loving feelings for a perpetrator destroys their vision of the innocence of children and childhood.

The child who struggles with intellectual or physical difficulties also challenges our images of childhood and often the child's identity is swamped by the diagnosis 'Jane is autistic' rather than 'Jane likes watching football'. The focus of help for all these children can be to repair rather than to accept and love the person in the present. So Alice, now 14, thought she was not acceptable to her adopted family for four years because it took her that long to be 'repaired'. We changed her narrative by helping her talk about the difficulties of understanding rules in families rather than coming to a new family because she was 'bad' and needed to become 'good'.

In pretend play and children's narratives 'monsters' mostly represent adults who have power and control over the children. It is interesting for adults to hear children's stories about their perceptions of monsters and perhaps share some stories in return. Some stories offer strategies to cope with 'monsters'. Sometimes we surrender to their demands, like Teeny-Tiny, at other times we can employ other strategies to cope. The role of adults is to attune to the child in play and talk, to respond carefully to what is said, to praise creativity and, as with Alice, to help the child reframe any distortions to enhance self-esteem.

Family monsters, past and present

Ruth made up the following three stories between the ages of four and five. She was fostered at the time, and waiting to find a permanent family. Ruth is trying to come to terms with the fact that her mother's drinking had meant that she couldn't care for her children. Her mother was still drinking heavily and couldn't or did not want to stop. The first story expresses some of the chaos of life when she was at home with her mother.

> Once upon a time there were two ducks.
> They were naughty.
> They bit themselves, got drunk,
> They shouted and everybody got scared.
> One duck was called Freddy.

He was drunk. He hit himself.
He hit everybody, himself, grown-ups
And children.
Then the grown-ups got drunk
And the children died.

The second story expresses Ruth's longing for her mother and her wish that she would come and see her children in a sober state. Ruth could accept her mother's drinking, what she called 'dirty drinking', but she needed a space in play to express the longing for mother to be sober.

The Cross Crocodile

Once upon a time a very cross crocodile
Smashed his teeth together shouting: 'I want my mum.'
Mum said, 'What are you doing?'
The crocodile said, 'What are you doing here, Mum? What are you doing in the room?'
'I have come just for a play.'
Today Mum is being sensible
Not being drunk
So she could look after crocodile, she could, she could.

In the third story Ruth is thinking about a new mum and dad and a peaceful place for herself and a new family.

The Lake Story

Once upon a time there was a lake.
It is nice and warm.
The dinosaurs live in the lake.
They drink the lake.
Everybody drinks out of the lake.
But it is not bad drink.
It is good drink like a milk shake.
It is pink.
The mummy dinosaur is singing.
She likes it.

These stories are very important for children in that state of limbo waiting for a new family, and carers need to attune to such narrations. These are moments when the child needs nurture and adults to support their hopes and dreams for a better future. It is important to tell the truth to children in a sensitive way and acknowledge their yearnings and dreams without promising what is not possible. Stuart, aged four, described his dream family:

Stuart's Story

There is a boy called Stuart,
He is four. He is good.
He has a mum and dad.
He goes to school.
He has a dog and a cat.
His mum and dad are good.
They look after him.
They don't get drunk.
They make good food.
And make sure he goes to school.

John is 12 and in foster care. He has ambivalent feelings about families and, like many children who feel ambivalent about parents, he has a yearning to be alone but with friends. Many children struggling with family life say they want to live by themselves when they are older. It seems less difficult than coping with moving and fitting in with yet another set of people.

Sid the Bird

Sid is a young bird,
He can fly somehow.
There was a bird called Sid.
He was young and he lived in between two trees.
The trees were near water.
It is quite warm.
He likes it there.
He has a mum and dad.
They are looking for food.
He still lives with them.
His best friend is a magpie called Alison.
They are playmates, just friends.
Sid's parents are reliable.
Their nest is beside the tree.
They stay close but not in the same nest.
Sid would like more birds to be his friends.

He gets lonely.
He does lots of coming and going.
He would like to be settled.
He wants to be left alone
Without Mum and Dad.
Maybe some more birds.

When children have ambivalent feelings about their parents a story can help. The story of *The Wicked Step-mother* from Togo, West Africa, ends with the step-mother admitting her cruelty, which is satisfying for many children.

The Wicked Step-mother

There was once a certain man who had two wives. The first one bore him a boy child and the other had no children.

Now it came to pass that the mother of the boy took sick, and when she knew that death was near she sent for the second wife and placed her in charge of her son saying, 'Take him and care for him and feed him as if he was your own.' The second wife agreed and shortly after the first wife died.

But the second wife forgot her promise and was very cruel to the boy. She gave him nether food nor clothing and the poor boy had to scavenge for himself.

One day the wife called the boy to her and said he must accompany her to the bush to get firewood.

The boy obeyed and went with the woman.

When they were a long way from the village the woman went into the bush for sticks and the boy sat down in the shade of a big tree. Presently he noticed a lot of fruit had fallen from the tree and he began to eat it.

He was very hungry and only when he had eaten all the fallen fruit was his hunger satisfied. He then fell asleep and after a while he woke and he was hungry again. But there was no fruit on the ground and he was far too small to reach up to the branches to gather some fruit. So the boy began to sing and as he sang a song in praise of the tree an amazing thing happened. The branches of the tree bent down to the boy and enabled him to climb up. He then took all the fruit he could eat and collected some to take home. Then still singing he climbed down and waited for the woman. She soon came and they both went home.

Some days later the boy was seated outside the house eating the fruit he had gathered. The woman saw him and asked him what he had there. He told her and the woman took some and said the fruit was really tasty. She then told the boy to go with her to the tree so they could get more of the new and excellent fruit.

They went and when they got near the tree the boy began to sing again and the tree obediently bent down its branches. And the woman climbed up. Then the boy ceased his singing and the branches sprang up taking the woman with them.

The woman now called to the boy but he answered that Nyame had now given him sense and shown him how to get food. And that as she had neglected him so now he would neglect her. He then went home to the village.

Now when he got home all the people asked him where was the woman. And he replied that she had gone into the bush to collect firewood.

Evening came and still no woman. So the people assembled under the village tree and again asked the boy. But he replied as before.

On the following morning the villagers again assembled and began to beg the boy to show them where he had left his step-mother. They begged and begged and at last he told them and led them into the bush where the people saw the woman at the top of the tree. They asked her how she had managed to get there and she told them. Then they all begged the boy to sing.

For a long time he refused. But at last they begged him so long he agreed. And began to sing his praise to the tree. Immediately the branches bent down and the woman was freed.

Then everyone went back to the village and reported to the chief what they had seen. He at once called all the elders and sent for the woman. He told her that had the boy not consented to sing she would not have been rescued and he ordered her to give an account of how she had treated the motherless child. She confessed she had done wrong and the chief said, 'Now let all men know from this that all children should be treated kindly by step-parents as well.'

This story of a monster step-mother is satisfying because the boy gains power over her and only he can control what happens to her. He frees her from the imprisonment in the tree and she admits her cruelty. It is interesting to ask the listening child what kind of relationship the boy and his step-mother might have in the future and how they might be reconciled and live together again. And where is his father? What is he doing to support his son?

New families, old fears

Hansel and Gretel

Close to a large forest there lived a woodcutter with his wife and his two children. The boy was called Hansel and the girl Gretel. The family was very poor, and now there was famine in the land and they could find nothing to eat.

The woodcutter was distraught and said to his wife, 'What is to become of us? How are we to feed our poor children when we have nothing for ourselves?'

'I'll tell you what, husband,' said the wife. 'Tomorrow morning, we will take the children out into the thickest part of the forest. We will light a fire and give each of them a piece of bread; then we will go out to work, and leave them alone. They won't be able to find their way back, so we shall be rid of them.'

The woodcutter said he could never find it in his heart to leave the children in the forest, but his wife gave him no peace until he consented.

'But I grieve over the poor children all the same,' said the woodcutter.

Children who move to new families and children who feel they don't fit in fear abandonment if they don't learn to conform. They remember what happened in the past and fear it will happen to them again and again. If they don't learn the rules in their new family will they be pushed out again? Why were they rejected in the first place? What do you have to do to be loveable so that adults will care for you?

Jade, aged five, has mixed feelings about her new parents. She loves the food, her bedroom, cuddles, but not the endless rules. She thinks her new mum is bossy, sometimes a witch and sometimes a lovely mum. The witch mum is a mixture of birth mum and new mum and Jade is not sure about the new mum. She fears being dumped again 'with no mum to look after them'.

Jade's Story

Once upon a time there was a witch.
She was a horrible witch.
She had no children because she was bad.
She turned them into frogs.
So the frog children jumped into the river
And they go all the way to London.
They had no mum to look after them
Because the witch was unkind to them.
In London they found a new mum and dad,
Not witches, just nice people.
They gave the children food, toys and a house,
Their own beds, a dog, a pussycat,
Hugs and kisses.
The End.

Jade found it difficult to trust adults to care for her. She remembered her mother's cruelty. She remembered moving from carer to carer. She liked to be soothed with a story which could give her hope for the future. There are many Cinderella stories from around the world, and Jade was fond of the following story which expressed her yearning for a loving adult who would care for her. It soothed her and she liked to hear it again and again. The right story which touches a child can create a bond between adult and child and become part of a family ritual or a connection between a professional worker and the child to define their relationship.

The Girl Who Went through Fire, Water and the Golden Gate

A man and wife had an only child and she was a girl. This girl was loved by her father and hated by her mother.

When the girl was eight years old her father died, and then her mother thought she would revenge herself on the girl. She made her do all the hard work in the house, and gave her many cruel tasks.

One day the mother sent the girl to fetch something that lay beyond three fields that were bewitched. When the child came to the first field she saw that it was covered with fire and she stood still at the edge of the field and dared not cross over it.

As she stood there trembling with fear and crying a beautiful fairy appeared to her and said, 'Don't be afraid. I will help you.' The fairy waved her wand across the field of fire. And the fire went out and the child went over.

But after she had gone a little way further on her way she came to a field which was covered with water and couldn't get across.

Then the beautiful fairy came near to her again as she wept and waved her wand over the water which rolled back on either side so that she walked straight through the middle.

So she went on her way again until she came to a house with a golden gate which she couldn't open or get through.

Then as before the fairy came with her wand and opened the gate, and when she opened the gate she said to the child, 'Leave your cruel mother and come and live with me.'

And the child said, 'Yes I will live with you for you are good and beautiful.'

So she left her cruel mother and went to live with the good fairy in the house with the golden gate.

Teachers as monsters

Sir is kind and sir is gentle,
Sir is strong and sir is mental.

God made the bees
The bees make honey
We do the work
And the teachers get the money.

A diller, a dollar,
A diller, a dollar,
A ten o'clock scholar,
What makes you come so soon?
You used to come at ten o'clock
And now you come at noon.

Like the ten o'clock scholar Sam, aged six, was reluctant to go to school. He felt sick every day before breakfast.

Sam says:
I am a bad boy.
I do naughty behaviour.
I am talking all the time.
Wriggling.
Not doing work.
Shouting.
Not listening to the teacher.
Cheeky to the teacher.
Fighting with the children.

Teacher says I must:
Listen then do as I am told.
Do my work.
Sit quietly.
No fighting.
No punching.
Stop being annoying.

Sam is struggling with his new adoptive family. Before being placed he lived in 12 foster homes. School is confusing for Sam, who has had to learn so many rules as he moved from family to family and school, and his somewhat punitive teacher is the final monster in a long line of monster adults. Nothing positive in the teacher's list, no warm praise for effort, just reinforcing his own view that he is a 'bad boy'. No wonder he feels sick every day.

McCartney (2007) states that children in our care system have an appalling record of educational achievement, and are ten times more likely to face exclusion from school. They frequently report feeling isolated and unloved. Simpson (2000) believes that the underlying intent of the school curriculum which orders the spatial and temporal lives of children is to ensure that schools are inhabited by 'docile bodies'. Childhood is seen as a period of control and passivity, during which the child's body is 'finished' and admitted into adult society. School rules dictate how students should comport themselves and part of the control exercised in schools is aimed at maintaining the correct use of space.

Rules such as:

- obey instructions/follow directions
- no shouting out or speaking without permission
- keep your hands, feet and objects to yourself
- stay in your seat unless you have permission to move
- no chewing

are very difficult for impulsive children who need to move about at intervals or children who have developmental difficulties with short concentration spans and anxiety about learning. So pity the teacher who has to engage with the rules and the children who have to try to keep them. No wonder the teacher sometimes becomes a monster. Teachers have limited training about managing distressed children who react badly to power battles. Creative thinking is required in a busy classroom to facilitate the learning of children who find such an environment stressful. There are many imaginative ways to support children and help them find their way in the school setting. Respect is a good start.

John, aged 12, described nine people turned to stone but only the teacher stayed stone for ever and ever. John was struggling at school and his teacher humiliated him by glaring at him and making personal remarks, which meant that he became the butt of his classmates' jokes. He could forgive many things but not the public humiliation. At least he could freeze her out in his story.

The Black Deadly Tree

The black deadly tree exists in some dark dark wood,
It is deadly because every time someone looks at it
It turns them to stone.
It has turned nine people to stone
And they are stuck around the tree.

1. Eddy because he came to cut down the tree.
2. Shona because she has been a horrible teacher.
3. Chris. He is a filthy man.
4. Martin because he was lobbing things at the deadly tree.
5. Lesley because she was shouting at the tree.
6. Fiona because she was swearing at the tree. 'You bastard.'

7. Bill because he was kicking the tree.
8. Frankenstein because he was cutting the tree down.
9. Superman because he was trying to freeze the tree with his superpowers.

Someone managed to unfreeze Superman.
He built a shield round himself so when the deadly tree was trying to freeze him it bounced off him onto the tree.
They managed to cut the tree down and saved everyone.
All eight people still frozen came unfrozen
Except for one person, the teacher.
She stayed there for ever and ever
And everyone managed to get out with their lives
Except the one person
Who was gawping at everyone.

Some children feel put down because they are not as clever as their classmates. I tell them the story of *The Two Foxes.*

The Two Foxes

A man was one day walking along the road with a creel of herrings on his back. And two foxes see him.

And the one who was biggest said to the other, 'Stop here and follow the man and I will run around and pretend that I am dead.'

So he ran around and stretched himself on the road.

The man came on and when he saw the fox he was well pleased to find so fine a beast. And he picked him up and threw him into the creel and went on.

Then the fox threw the herrings out of the creel and the other followed and picked them up. And when the creel was empty the big fox jumped out and ran away and that was how they got the herrings.

Well, they went on together until they came to the Smith's house.

And there was a horse tied at the door. And he had a golden shoe and there was a name on it.

'I will go and read what is written on that shoe,' said the big fox and he went.

But the horse lifted his foot and struck a kick on him and drove his brains out.

'Lad, lad,' said the little fox, 'no scholar me nor wish I to be.'
And of course he got the herrings.

Doctors as monsters *by Alison Webster*

Alison Webster is a play therapist and a hospital play services manager.
She describes children's responses to healthcare and the paradoxes of
adults who heal people but in the process cause physical pain to the child.

Play-based narratives within healthcare

There is a story I read in my childhood called *Marianne Dreams* by
Catherine Storr (1958) which is a narrative on illness involving two
school-age children, both with infectious diseases. One child, Marianne,
is being cared for at home, another requires invasive medical treatment in
hospital. Both children face long recovery periods, with prolonged
periods of confinement and isolation.

The story involves use of a magic pencil, which, through use of
Marianne's imagination, gives the possibility of freedom. Her drawings
seem to provide her a fantasy world of release from the day-to-day
frustrations of illness, confinement and boredom – but which fast
becomes a world full of unexplained fears, of being watched, entrapped
and potentially annihilated. The child Marianne creates as a companion
within this world becomes part of a narrative which unfolds to reveal that
this other child, a boy, is in hospital in an iron lung. He describes being
watched by nurses and doctors and his parents for signs of getting better
or worse.

Boundaries between dream and waking worlds start to blur and bleed
into one another with consequences for both children as they seek to
regain their health and the normality of their lives. Marianne asks a
question central to many children's experiences of illness: 'How did we
get here and why is everything outside so horrible? What are *they*
watching us for? What are *they* waiting for?' (p.114).

Children under the age of five are particularly vulnerable to
healthcare, specifically due to their limited verbal skills and fears around
being separated from their significant carers. But older children also have
anxieties within healthcare, some of which may go undetected by staff
due to an assumption made that these children will be better able to use

verbal skills to cope with their experiences and in getting their needs met. Little research has been done into how children build both their under-standing of stressful events and their coping repertoires. This has an impact on our assessment of how children cope with stress and regression caused by illness, plus that of the effects of the hospital environment.

Power relationships between patient and medical worlds are rarely considered – particularly when thinking about the needs of dis-empowered children who are so dependent on adults. I have often had said to me both implicitly and explicitly that 'we haven't time' when I advocate a child-centred approach which incorporates a dialogue based on play philosophies; that is, not just the aural, verbally based adult language which can serve to distance children from adults as well as adults from children.

Table 6.1 represents a variety of developmental play which supports children's needs within healthcare. It is a general overview of suggestions but out of which may evolve imaginative and therapeutic narratives, which a sensitive adult can support as co-constructed dialogue with a child.

Story-telling as part of the healing process

When I consider the narratives which both children and adults in healthcare construct to help make sense of what is happening around them, such as why a child has to have medical treatment, and why an adult has to inflict pain as part of this process, it is how we share our stories which offers perhaps the most beneficial aspect of healing and empower-ment for both groups. The feelings aroused around these potentially difficult experiences of healthcare are very real for all parties concerned, and in my professional opinion can mirror some of the feelings that you might better expect to see arise in the play of troubled children who have been abused. It is not unrealistic to suggest a further parallel from which to consider the feelings of medical staff who 'perpetrate' pain as a part of invasive care which has to be given. Perhaps it is understandable why such staff, without appropriate support, may over-distance themselves emotionally from the children they seek to care for.

Table 6.1: Suggestions to enable adults and children to reconnect through play

Type of play	Babies	School age	Teenagers
Tactile, sensory play e.g. rattles, teethers, cot and activity centres, mobiles, fibre optic toys, stress balls	Very important that all equipment meets safety standards and is maintained. Black and white toys helpful for visual stimulation of very young babies. Bright, easily washable toys useable in floor play, by the bedside and in pushchairs or when being held, e.g. during treatment, are helpful.	This age group often likes to explore sensory toys, but may feel embarrassed as they consider them too babyish. Use of specialist toys such as fibre optics often gets over this concern. Such toys can help relax a child, e.g. before, during and after treatment.	Use of stress balls is particularly helpful for this age group and will also recognize those teenagers who may have special needs and could benefit from tactile play support to raise their coping skills with treatment and as an aid to relaxation.
Soft toys e.g. teddies, etc.	These can be comforting – especially if it is a favourite teddy etc. from home. Sometimes a baby will have a 'comfort blanket' in place of this, or a soother. It is important to find out if there is such a comforter as this will help in any stressful situations. Due to infection controls we generally use the child's teddy etc. or a specialized supply of soft toys only used as part of our play preparation programme. Any secondhand donations must be disposed of safely.	Soft toys can be very useful for giving emotional support – and the fact that many are animals is important, as they are removed from reality to some degree. They can be used to help a child play out their feelings and voice unspoken concerns or anxieties.	A common side effect of illness is regression – going back to earlier patterns of behaviour. Teenagers can sometimes seem to find some comfort through a soft toy – especially if it is an old childhood favourite. They should never be made to feel embarrassed about such needs.

Home/role-play e.g. kitchen corner, medical toy sets, dressing-up clothes	Children as young as a year old can enjoy simple toys familiar from home such as a toy tea set – such play supporting a range of co-ordination, social, imaginative and emotional needs.	Home corners need to reflect the diversity of the cultures of the children playing with them, e.g. tea-sets, balti and wok sets, plus suggestions of food from varied countries, dressing-up clothes, and also options to change the area into, e.g., an office or hospital are important to consider.	Medical play tends to be the predominant form of role-play support for this age group within the hospital setting, using a range of real equipment appropriate to needs.
Arts and crafts e.g. painting, drawing, sticking and collage	Very simple feet and hand painting involving the parents can be very helpful for this age group – as much benefit to the family sometimes! It is important to ensure adequate planning for such activities as they will require constant supervision.	This age group are often particularly interested in this area of play and quickly become motivated and involved in display and project work as it is so familiar from school life. Be sensitive to cultural needs and try to ensure this is reflected in the choice of themes in such play. Make sure that you do not 'take over' such play and give time and space for children to work at their own pace, with support offered when necessary.	Teenagers may need encouragement to participate and should never be put under pressure to do so – but if willing to engage, can often show great enjoyment and a variety of skills. It is important to remember not to concentrate on artistic ability, but rather on making the activity enjoyable. Again caution must be taken in over-interpretation. Observing developmental skills without being obtrusive can be useful during such activities.

Continued on next page

Table 6.1 continued

Type of play	Babies	School age	Teenagers
Messy play e.g. clay, Play Doh, water, sand, plasticine	Preparation is all! Make sure that you have all you need to safely supervise such play. Babies often enjoy water play and blowing bubbles – or using messy play such as corn flour 'slime' as an extension of tactile play which can be very limited by illness and medical care. N.B. Be aware that such play can raise anxieties – especially if families are uncomfortable with it, e.g. due to a cultural reason.	Often viewed as an 'antidote' to clinical aspects of the child's care in hospital, this type of play seems to have particular value in helping children talk about their feelings and how they feel about their bodies. Anger, resentment and the need to make a mess can all be channelled very constructively into these activities.	Using this medium of play can be helpful in enabling other members of the multidisciplinary team to work with all ages – and can be helpful in motivating, e.g., teenagers to complete physio exercises, as co-ordination and movement are integral to much of the enjoyment to be gained from such activities. N.B. All messy play must be supervised at all times.
Stories e.g. reading corner with a collection of fairy tales, everyday tales, hospital stories, etc.	Simple, repetitive and familiar stories can be very helpful in supporting normal routines, e.g. bed time and the parent–child relationship.	For the child who is old enough to distinguish between fantasy and reality, stories can provide a valuable resolution of inner conflicts and anxiety. A child will often identify with a character and use them as a non-threatening means to help overcome fears, uncertainties and as a way to voice their own problems.	Careful selection of reading materials is necessary to support all ages – paying particular attention to cultural aspects, equality and inclusion of modern themes relevant to an older age group.

Music

e.g. tapes from home, multicultural CDs, music sessions for groups of children, instruments for children in isolation or when bed bound

Playing music can be helpful for a number of reasons:

- It can help distract and comfort a wide age range of babies, children and teenagers.

- It can help mask highly clinical sounds from the hospital environment.

- It can calm families and support them as they interact with their child – especially when used as part of a sensory play or relaxation session.

- It can encourage younger children to move and dance, increasing confidence and aiding in the recovery of lost skills, e.g. after surgery.

- It can provide links with home and family culture.

- Playing an instrument can provide a direct and satisfying relationship between the child and their actions – particularly useful for children with special needs. The child can feel a sense of control over their environment.

- Music can take the place of words and sounds that a child may find difficult or feel unable to use.

Examples of children's narratives in healthcare

Many children use monsters in their stories while working with me to help provide a safe distance to acknowledge, explore and process their feelings about medical staff inflicting uncomfortable, sometimes painful and distressing treatments on them. It is easy to assume here that I talk only of obviously difficult treatments such as those involving needles. For many children it is also procedures that are strange but not necessarily painful or invasive that can cause just as much distress.

JANE'S NARRATIVES

Jane was 18. She was overwhelmed by her fear of an X-ray scanner used regularly to track her health needs. She would mask this fear with anger, using destructive avenues such as non-compliance with her diabetic care. She used her play therapy to develop many story themes around 'Pandora's Box', where she lifted the lid (both metaphorically and literally using a sand box) to build a complex world peopled by monsters, devils and angels as she tried to gain a better sense of 'Who in the world am I – who can I go to when I need help?'

ALAN'S NARRATIVES

Alan was a 16-year-old boy with disabilities. He narrated the following story around his doctor and his and his family's anger after an out-patients consultation around a medical situation which remained unresolved at this point in time:

> My doctor is angry. Because he doesn't know what to do – doesn't know why everybody is standing there. He wants to be a monster – to kick everybody over. The nurses go up to him and ask what the matter is. He says, 'I don't know what to do.' His car is there just in case he needs a fast get away from all the other people because they're giving him a hard time...This is my doctor going on holiday like he always does. And this is the grave digger – because he has to dig the graves of everyone that's died.

The theme of monsters seemed to centre on how this boy viewed his doctor's frustrations, but was also perhaps a projection of the boy's own feelings of anger at the time towards the doctor, which he felt able to express through the safety of symbolic play. The clarity of vision which he shared with me over the lifelong impact of his health needs was poignant, as was the acknowledgement of his fear of death and the intrinsic part his doctor played in his life. In line with his developmental stage, this boy was able to take a far more abstract view of his situation and his awareness of just how frustrated he understood his doctor to be in making the right decisions about his ongoing care was truly insightful, as many staff did not consider him capable of understanding a great deal of the details around his healthcare needs.

Another young person disclosed a horror of speaking to his doctors due to seeing them as 'horrible, scary – I'm afraid of them and I don't want to get on their wrong side'. He was eventually able to communicate with his doctors through use of a dictaphone, which he used in his play therapy to help confront his unrecognized fear of being misunderstood by the medical team. Slowly he was able to ask important questions and voice his concerns using these narratives, which contained his fear, 'humanizing' his understanding of his doctors through this process. I acted as a mediator using transcriptions of our work to help clarify his needs to the medical team and his family without this child being overwhelmed by either his or their anxiety.

The following stories were told to me by Andrea, an 11-year-old girl with a chronic health condition and experiences of many hospital admissions from birth.

The Adventure Maze

[…]two green monsters had taken the treasure…The monsters knew Max, Sam and Johnny were going to the maze – they had overheard – the boys weren't scared at first because they didn't recognize the monsters. But then one monster started to follow them…they were very scared and were trapped. The manager came into the maze looking for the monsters – he could hear screaming and saw the monsters trapping the boys. 'I thought I'd told you to stop scaring people – now get out!' he said. He took the masks and costumes off the monsters and then the boys saw that they weren't real monsters – they were the bullies…

A second story shortly after this session went as follows:

The Playground

This is an animal adventure playground – it is a crèche for the younger kids – they like it here because of the toys and that their parents aren't there. But they didn't have a choice. The children felt lonely and rejected... One little boy is terrified of all the creepy crawlies looking at him and nobody playing with him... Everyone left to go home. The two ladies who look after the crèche remembered the little boy – but they had trouble opening the gate... The boy was shaking and he ran into a tunnel because he was scared of the animals that might eat him. The boy thought the ladies were monsters so he didn't make a sound. But he started to cry and the ladies found him in the tunnel. 'I thought it was the monsters!' he cried... He felt relieved.

Analysing these stories made for interesting discussions with Andrea. She was quite clear that the maze she refers to in her first story was 'like the hospital – you never know where you are and get lost easily'. Her drawing also showed a maze with an entrance but no way out through its convolutions – this theme of entrapment and lack of escape being another common theme recurring in many children's narratives. Considering the monsters in the maze, I wondered who they might

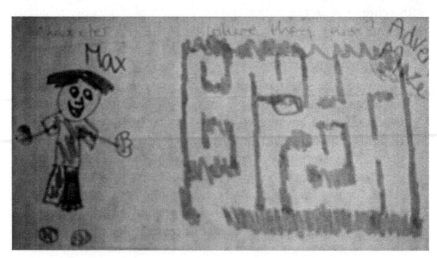

A write and draw method to help an 11-year-old engage with story telling in an age appropriate way

represent – whether the bullying theme they linked with might be connected with school? Bullying is a very common difficulty many children who have a chronic health condition face – so might seem to be the obvious meaning behind the story. Again the child was very clear with me that she thought the monsters were the anaesthetists and surgeons she had so often had to cope with over the years – which makes sense when you consider the aspects of disguise and masks contained within her story. This was perhaps the first time that Andrea had been able to openly acknowledge her anger and feelings of being bullied by these staff; also of feeling lost and abandoned by her family – left to face whatever 'monsters there might be in the maze' by herself (the reality of this situation being that there had to be short, usually overnight periods when the child's mother went home due to work and other family commitments).

It is within this arena of feelings that play can be a powerful medium whereby the adult and the child can meet creatively, can challenge, listen and value one another within a narrative structure which encourages understanding and empowers the child. Based on my own experience as both practitioner and manager of specialist play programmes, it takes courage on behalf of all concerned to face the 'monsters' that may lie waiting.

The self as monster

Many children blame themselves for all the difficulties they have experienced and so define themselves as monsters. Sam who tried so hard to be 'good' at school blames himself saying he is 'naughty'. Janice loved to draw and I gave her two plain white papier-mâché masks of faces. She decorated them and told the following stories about the masks. Janice is perceptive about herself as she struggles to find joy and self-regard.

The Family Mask

The mask is called Fred Frustration.
This is a male mask.
The lips are red and wide.
It is a forced smile.
The eyelashes are clear and controlled.
The tears are messy.

One cheek is the sun.
The sun is half out, half formed.
The sun is waiting.
The sunshine girl is overshadowed by the dad.
He won't leave her alone.
He keeps picking on her.
The other cheek is a silver cloud.
It's made of soft rock.
You can't eat it.
The rock under the cloud is squashed.
Maybe squashed for ever.
Maybe not.
Lost half the chance to have other suns.
Confusion shows in tears.
The top of the head is red.
It is angry curls.
Shouting screaming.
Glad to be live.
Don't want to be dead.
There is a chance for the sun to come out.
Don't know how to do that.

Mask of the Genitals

Whole of my body.
My body is ugly.
Unhappy.
Mouth really unhappy.
Acid tears.
But also acid everything that leaves the body.
If somebody touches my tears they get burnt
Embarrassed.
Tacky bits of my body.
Embarrassed.
Whole of my body.
My body is ugly.
Unhappy.
Mouth really unhappy.
Everything sunk in.
Don't want anyone to look.
It is about shame.

Shame about what happened.
To find some pleasure in my body.
How to change is a puzzle.
When my brother abused me,
It felt sneaky.
Body like an animal
Drips green slime
Has wings, can fly.
Poor sight.

Stories about managing monsters

I enjoy the story of *Nuckelavee* because it has such a gruesome monster, pulsating flesh and no skin. Tammas escapes because the monster is afraid of fresh water. So often monsters have a secret fear which is their undoing once it is understood. I like Tammas's final exhausted leap across the fresh water stream to safety leaving his hat in the monster's arms. Tammas is no great hero, just an ordinary man in danger who manages his fear and escapes. Nuckelavee lives to find other victims and Tammas lives to tell his story.

Nuckelavee

Nuckelavee was a frightening evil monster who never rested from his evil ways. He lived in the sea and when he was there he moved through the seas as if by magic.

When he came on land he rode a horse which looked as frightening as Nuckelavee.

Some people thought that the rider and the horse were really one and that this was the shape of the monster.

Nuckelavee's head was like a man's only ten times larger and his mouth stuck out like a pig's mouth. It was huge and wide. There was not a hair on the monster for the very good reason that he had no skin.

If the crops were destroyed by the sea-gust, if cattle fell over the rocks into the sea or if men became ill with strange fevers, Nuckelavee was the cause of it all. His breath was poison, falling like a deadly disease on animals and crops. He was blamed for causing droughts. He had serious objections to fresh water and was never known to visit the land during rain.

This is the story of a man called Tammas who once encountered Nuckelavee and had a narrow escape from the monster's clutches.

Tammas was out late one night. It was a fine starlit night. Tammas's road lay close to the sea-shore and as he entered a part of the road that was hemmed in on one side by the sea and the other by a deep fresh-water loch he saw some huge object in front of and moving towards him. What was he to do?

He was sure it was no earthly thing that was coming towards him. He could not go to either side and to turn his back on an evil thing was the most dangerous position of all. Tammas was always regarded as rough and foolish. Anyway he decided as the better of two evils to face the foe and move resolutely forward. Then he discovered that the evil thing moving towards him was no other than the dreaded Nuckelavee.

The lower part of the monster was like a great horse with flappers like fins around its legs. It had a mouth as wide as a whale and its breath was like a steaming kettle. It had one eye and that was red as fire. On him sat or seemed to grow from his back a huge man with no legs and arms that reached nearly to the ground. His huge head kept rolling from one shoulder to the other as if it meant to tumble off.

But what to Tammas appeared most horrible of all was that the monster was skinless. The whole surface of its body showed only red raw flesh in which Tammas saw blood black as tar running through yellow veins and great white sinews twisting and stretching as the monster moved.

Tammas was terrified, his hair stood on end and cold sweats came from every pore. But he knew it was useless to flee and he would rather face the monster if he were to die.

Although he was terrified Tammas remembered that Nuckelavee was afraid of fresh water so he took that side of the road nearest the fresh water loch.

The most terrifying moment came when the lower part of the head of the monster got abreast of Tammas.

The mouth of the monster appeared like a pit, the hot breath felt like fire in his face. The monster's long arms stretched out to grab Tammas.

Tammas swerved towards the loch. In doing so one of his feet went into the loch splashing up some fresh water on the foreleg of the monster. The monster gave a snort-like thunder and staggered to the side of the road.

Tammas saw his opportunity and ran as fast as he could. Nuckelavee galloped after him bellowing like the roaring of the ocean.

In front of Tammas lay a small stream through which the surplus water in the loch found its way to the sea. And Tammas knew if he could cross the stream he was safe. The monster was clutching at Tammas who made a desperate leap across the stream, leaving his hat in the monster's clutches.

Nuckelavee gave a wild unearthly yell of disappointed rage as Tammas fell exhausted on the safe side of the water.

Li Chi Slays the Serpent is a story about a young girl who is brave and clever enough to slay the monster. The story is set in a time and culture when girls were considered to be useless, worthless and a burden to the family yet, paradoxically, this young girl, Li Chi, is loved by her parents, is brave and strong and ends by killing the serpent and marrying the king. This paradox of being strong but at the same time feeling worthless is still the struggle of many young women as they try to find a place for themselves in the family and at school.

Li Chi Slays the Serpent

In Fukien Province stand the Yung Mountains whose peaks sometimes reach a height of many miles. To the north west there is a gap in the mountains once inhabited by a giant serpent 70 or 80 feet long and wider than ten hand spans.

The people were terrified of this snake and it had already killed many people including important officers from the nearby towns. Offerings of animals did not satisfy the monster who sent messages to the people through entering men's dreams. The monster demanded young girls of 12 and 13 to feast on.

Helpless the town commander and the magistrates selected daughters of servants or criminals and kept them for the serpent. One day in the eighth month of every year they would deliver a girl to the mouth of the monster's cave and the serpent would come out and swallow the victim. This continued for nine years until nine girls had been devoured.

In the tenth year the officials again began looking for a girl to appease the monster's appetite. A man from Chianglo Province called Li Tan had raised six daughters and no sons. Li Chi, his youngest girl, responded to the search for a victim by volunteering. Her parents refused to allow it but Li Chi said that as they had no sons to support the family she could give a little money to the family to help them and she wouldn't be a burden to them in the future.

But her parents loved Li Chi too much to agree to her offer. So Li Chi went in secret.

She then asked the officials for a sharp sword and a snake-hunting dog. When the day of the sacrifice arrived she seated herself in the temple clutching the sword and leading the dog. First she took several piles of rice balls moistened with malt sugar and placed them at the mouth of the serpent's cave.

The serpent appeared. Its head was as large as a rice barrel. Its eyes were like mirrors two feet across.

Smelling the fragrance of the rice balls it opened its mouth to eat them. Then Li Chi unleashed the snake-hunting dog which bit hard into the serpent. Li Chi herself came behind the dog and slashed the serpent with her sword scoring several deep cuts. The serpent screamed in pain and leapt out of its cave and died.

Li Chi went into the cave and recovered the skulls of the nine victims. She sighed as she brought them out saying, 'You were so fearful that the serpent destroyed you. How sad. What a waste.'

The king heard of Li Chi's bravery and married her. Her family were given riches. From that time the district was free from monsters and the exploits of Li Chi are celebrated to this day.

Peace from the monsters

David was ten when he told this story. He has clever strategies to escape from the monster. David's family life had been full of monsters, his father and his mother's boyfriend were both abusive and both violent. David had learnt many ways to avoid attention so that he wouldn't be threatened and hurt by these men. Being invisible was what he wanted for himself and that yearning for a safe haven without the threat of other people.

David's Monster

It's a silent monster.
Makes no sound.
Runs fast.
David runs and runs.
The monster chases silently.
David gets to a wall.
No way out.
Trapped.
The monster can fly
But it can only see red.
So if David is dressed in black
Or throws off any red clothing
Then he becomes invisible.
The monster would try to look
But wouldn't find David.
When the monster is gone
David quietly flies away.
To a hot country.
On the beach
With the sea lapping
Just alone
To sleep.

I told David the story of *The Two Mice*. After so much fear there is a yearning to be soothed, to find peace and quiet from a cruel world.

The Two Mice

There was a mouse on the hill, and a mouse on a farm.
   'It were well,' said the hill mouse, 'to be on the farm, where one might get things.'
   Said the farm mouse, 'Better is peace.'

CHAPTER 7

Books and Stories that Mirror the Child's Life Experiences

Stories

These stories are all folk tales and have themes that may connect with some children's life experiences. The first story is a Tlingit (Native American) monster story with an interesting twist. The monster is killed but changes into a cloud of mosquitoes, forever sucking on humans. It could lead to talk with children about those painful reminders of hurt and abuse that remain as constant reminders of the past.

How Mosquitoes Came to Be

Long ago there was a giant who loved to kill people, eat their flesh and drink their blood. He was especially fond of human hearts. 'Unless we can get rid of this giant,' people said, 'none of us will be left.' And they called a council to discuss ways and means.

One man said, 'I think I know how to kill the monster,' and he went to the last place the giant had been seen. There he lay down and pretended to be dead. Soon the giant came along. Seeing the man lying there he said, 'These humans are making it easy for me. Now I don't even have to catch and kill them. They might die right on my trail probably from fear of me.' The giant touched the body.

'Ah good,' he said, 'this one is still warm and fresh. What a tasty meal he will make. I can't wait to get him home.'

The giant flung the man over his shoulder and the man let his head hang down as if he were dead. Carrying the man home the giant dropped him in the middle of the floor near the fireplace. Then he saw that there was no firewood so he went to get some.

As soon as the giant had left the man got up and grabbed the giant's huge skinning knife. Just then the giant's son came in, bending low to enter. He was still small as giants go and the man held the big knife to his throat. 'Quick, tell me where your father's heart is. Tell me or I'll slit your throat.'

The giant's son was scared. He said, 'My father's heart is in his left heel.'

Just then the giant's left foot appeared in the entrance and the man swiftly plunged the knife into the heel. The monster screamed and fell down dead.

Yet the giant still spoke. 'Although I am dead, though you killed me, I'm going to keep on eating you and all the other humans in the world for ever.'

'That's what you think,' said the man. 'I'm about to make sure that you never eat anyone ever again.'

He cut the giant's body into little pieces and burned each one in the fire. Then he took the ashes and threw them into the air for the winds to scatter. Instantly each of the particles turned into a mosquito. The cloud of ashes became a cloud of mosquitoes and from the midst the man heard the giant's voice laughing, saying, 'Yes, I'll eat you people until the end of time.'

And as the monster spoke the man felt a sting and a mosquito started sucking his blood and then many mosquitoes stung him and he began to scratch himself.

The second story, from Lebanon, describes a quick-thinking hero who, although not as strong as his brothers, is cleverer at getting out of trouble and is loyal to his family, rescuing his brothers from the hyena. So Little Mangy One is triumphant and I think needs a change of name.

Little Mangy One

Once upon a time three little goats were grazing on the side of a stony hill. Their names were Siksik, Mikmik and Jureybon, the Little Mangy One. Soon a hyena scented them and loped up.

'Siksik,' called the hyena.

'Yes sir,' answered the goat.

'What are those points sticking out of your head?'

'Those are my little horns, sir,' said the goat.

'What is that patch on your back?' continued the hyena.

'That is my hair, sir,' replied the goat.

'Why are you shivering?' roared the hyena.

'Because I am afraid of you, sir,' said the goat.

At this the hyena sprang and gobbled him right up.

Next the hyena turned to Mikmik who answered like his brother and he too was quickly devoured. Then the hyena approached Jureybon, the Little Mangy One.

Before the hyena came within earshot, Jureybon began to snort. As the hyena drew nearer Jureybon bellowed, 'May a plague lay low your back O Cursed One. What have you come for?'

'I wish to know what the two points in your head are for.'

'Those. Why those are my trusted sabres,' said the goat.

'And the patch on your back, what is that?' asked the hyena.

'My sturdy shield, of course,' sneered the goat.

'Then why are you shivering?' asked the hyena.

'Shivering? I'm trembling with rage. I'm shaking with impatience for I cannot wait to throttle you and squeeze your very soul till it starts out of your eye sockets,' snarled the goat, and began to advance on the hyena.

The hyena's heart stopped beating for a moment, then he turned and ran for his life. But Jureybon sprang after him over the rocks and gored him with his sharp little horns slitting open his belly and freeing his two little brothers inside.

There are many stories about the Wise Men of Gotham and this English one describes two men arguing over non-existent sheep. They are shown the error of their ways by another man of Gotham, who loses his sack of meal in the process, so who is the wisest? That's an interesting discussion. Similar stories are universal. There are 36 Irish versions, 52 Swedish and Russian, Hungarian, Indian and Indonesian stories to name but a few. This story is reminiscent of those circular arguments which go round and round with no capacity to solve problems.

The Wise Men of Gotham – Buying of Sheep

There were two men of Gotham and one of them was going to Nottingham market to buy sheep and the other came from the market and they both met together on Nottingham Bridge.

'Where are you going?' asked the one who came from Nottingham.

'Good day,' said he who was going to Nottingham. 'I am going to buy sheep.'

'Buy sheep?' said the other. 'And which way will you bring them home?'

'I will bring them over this bridge,' said the other.

'By Robin Hood,' said the man from Nottingham, 'but thou shall not.'

'By Maid Marion,' said the other, 'but I will.'

'You will not,' said the one.

'I will,' said the other.

Then they beat their sticks against the ground one against the other as if there were a hundred sheep between them.

'Hold in,' said the one, 'beware lest my sheep jump over the bridge.'

'I care not,' said the other. 'They shall not come this way.'

'But they shall,' said the other.

Then the other said, 'If you make much to do, I will put my fingers in your mouth.'

'Will you?' said the other.

Now, as they were arguing, another man from Gotham came from the market with a sack of meal upon a horse, seeing and hearing his neighbours arguing about sheep though there were no sheep there.

'Ah fools, will you ever learn wisdom? Help me and lay my sack upon my shoulders.'

They did so and he went to the side of the bridge, unloosed the mouth of the sack and shook all his meal out into the river.

'Now neighbours,' he said. 'How much meal is there in the sack?'

'Good heavens,' they said. 'There is none at all.'

'Now by my faith,' said he, 'even as much wit as is in your two heads to stir up strife about a thing you have not.'

Which was the wisest of these three persons? Judge yourself.

Another popular theme of folk tales is that of Jack the lad, sometimes clever, often the opposite, usually under the control of his mother. This is a story of Jack and his mother and, although Jack has a literal view of the world and can't adapt to new circumstances, in the end he finds companionship and a life with someone who is not irritated by his behaviour and finds fun in his antics. It takes all sorts to make a world. It is a story of hope and praise for difference.

Jack's Rewards and What He Did With Them

Jack was not too clever and when his father died his mother said he must go out to work but he could only do odd jobs. The first day he helped a peddler to carry his pack and the peddler gave him a needle. He carried it home in a bundle of hay and lost it. His mother said he should have stuck it in his cap.

The next day he carried some ploughs for the smith and was allowed to take some metal parts home. He put them in his cap but as he was leaning down to drink out of a stream they slipped in and were lost. 'You should have tied a string round them and pulled them behind you,' said his mother.

Next day he worked for a butcher who gave him a sheep's joint. He tied a string round it, pulled it behind him and there wasn't much left by the time he got home. 'You should have hung it over your shoulder,' said his mother.

The next day he worked with a horse cooper who gave him an old horse. He tied its legs together and tried to lift it but he couldn't, so he had to leave it by the roadside. 'You should have rode it back,' said his mother.

The next day he worked with a dairyman and did so well with the dairyman that the dairyman gave him an old cow. He got on its back. He didn't find it easy to ride but he got hold of its tail and steered it by that.

On the way he passed a rich gentleman's castle. The gentleman had a sad daughter, so sad that he had promised that any man who could make her laugh should marry her. When she saw Jack riding the cow and steering it by the tail she had to laugh and the gentleman sent his servant running after Jack to tell him he was to marry the lady.

They sent for Jack's mother to come to the wedding and they were all very happy. Jack was always slow but his antics kept his wife laughing all her life.

Mermaid stories are global and many describe the loss of family and environment experienced by the mermaid. In the Orkney story of *The Breckness Mermaid* the mermaid is torn between returning home to the sea and leaving behind the children she loves, although forced into marriage. In all these stories it is one of her children who facilitates the return to the sea by finding the mermaid's skin. There are many issues in such stories which connect to children removed from their families. Do you lose your skin when you leave your familiar home and environment? Will you always yearn for what is lost? Are you responsible for the loss of your mother? These stories also signify the loss of country, what it feels like to be 'out of your skin' and so relevant for refugees and others living in unfamiliar environments.

The Breckness Mermaid

One fine summer's day a Breckness man was walking along the shore. He was admiring the view of the breaking waves on the huge red cliffs of Hoy. The only sound was the cry of the seabirds which circled above his head and the sound of the waves hitting the rocks. He lay down on the beach and gazed at the ocean.

Then he saw the most beautiful sight he had ever seen. It was a mermaid bathing in the sea right in front of him. Her face was the most exquisite he had ever seen and her golden hair like spun gold. He had never seen such a wondrous creature and he fell in love immediately.

On the rock near to where the mermaid swam lay her sea skin. The young man knew if he could get possession of the skin the mermaid could not return to her home under the sea. She would be in his power and would have to follow him back home to his house.

He left the spot where he lay and crept towards the rock like a cat. The mermaid had left the sea and was combing her long golden hair. The man was so near to her now that he snatched the skin and hid it under his clothes. At that moment the mermaid saw him and turned to seize her skin but it was gone.

The tears rolled down her lovely face as she stared at the man who was the cause of her sorrows. She pleaded with him to give her back her skin so that she could return to the sea, but he refused. He wished her to come home with him to be his bride but she refused. After some time she finally agreed and they went home to his house.

They were married and lived together for a number of years. They had six fine children, three boys and three girls. The children were said to be the most beautiful children in Orkney. When they grew up their mother tried to get them to discover where their father kept her stolen sea skin. After being questioned about the skin for some time the man told his favourite daughter where he had hidden it. She ran to her mother delighted at her success in finding the information her mother wanted.

Soon after hearing the news the mermaid disappeared. Many long hours the man spent wandering the shore where he had first seen his mermaid wife but she was never there. The birds circled overhead as they had done on that first day but the mermaid did not come back to swim and comb her golden hair. One day the man was hiding behind some large rocks on the shore when he saw the mermaid come out of the sea. Her children ran down the shore to meet her and she sat and combed their hair. As soon as the man appeared she returned to the sea.

Many times she returned to that spot to comb the children's hair but she made sure that her sea skin was close by her hand.

It is said that if you go to the shore at Breckness you can still hear the sweet song of the mermaid. It was a lullaby to lull her children to sleep. The echoes of her song can never die but will forever drift around the rocks and waters of the deep.

I enjoy the mystery of the Orkney story of *The Lost Girl*. Where is she living or is she alive and who are her companions? Does she ever grow old? Again we feel the sense of loss as her father chooses a gold plate as a gift rather than asking for his daughter to return home with him. This theme is explored by J.M. Barrie, the author of *Peter Pan*, in his play *Mary*

Rose, about a young girl who disappears then returns, haunted by the past but unable to grow up.

The Lost Girl

There was once a family who lived in the North Isles, a father, a mother, two sons and a daughter. One day the daughter was sent to gather limpets for bait, but she never returned. Her family searched high and low but there was no sign of the girl.

Years later the father and two sons went fishing. It was a fine day when they left but soon it became foggy and they had no idea where they were or how to get home. After a while, the boat beached on an island shore. The three men left the boat and followed a path, which led to a beautiful home. They knocked on the door and it was answered by a handsome man. He invited them in saying they could stay until the fog cleared.

The men gasped at the sight of all the beautiful furnishings in the house, it was even grander than the king's house. The man introduced them to his wife who was none other than the lost girl. She welcomed her father and brothers warmly, asking after their health and all the folk back home. Her husband asked his father-in-law if he had any cattle to sell. He said that he did have one fine cow that he could have, and the man paid well for it in gold sovereigns. Now the old man thought that he could find out what island they were on. He said, 'Well, you'll have to tell me now how to get here or I'll not be able to take the cow to you.'

'Oh,' said the man, 'don't you worry about that – I'll come for the cow myself.'

One of the brothers said that the fog was lifting and they should be on their way. The girl said, 'Is there anything in the house that you would fancy to take home with you?' Her husband said, 'You're welcome to take anything that's here, just pick anything you would like and take it with you.' The girl gave them a hopeful look, thinking that her father would choose her. But his eye had fallen on a large gold plate and he took that home with him instead.

As they pushed the boat back down to the sea the man said, 'Just pull that way a bit.' And they headed into the bank of fog. As they came out the other side they found themselves near their own island. When they reached their home they found the old woman very agitated. 'An awful thing has happened. Our best cow is lying in the byre dead.' But the old man smiled and said, 'Ach let her go, she's well paid for.'

The island, the man and girl were never seen again.

The Girl That Couldn't Be Frightened is a Scottish story that defines girls as strong and capable of looking after themselves. There is also that desire to live alone which comes when parenting has been poor. The story also expresses the need to find another person who understands a weakness and describes how people can live together. You don't have to be a hero and strong all the time, but the girl's brave deeds are great fun.

The Girl That Couldn't Be Frightened

There was once a girl and nothing ever gave her a fright. At least that is what folks said about her. She lived all alone on a small farm in the middle of the forest. Her mother died when she was very small and her father – poor man – was never much use to her. He was more fond of a drink at the inn in the village nearby than being at home or at work. Besides that, one day he just wandered away somewhere and wherever it was he went he never came back. When it was plain to see he was gone for good folks told her she'd best come down to live in the village seeing she had no relations of her own to take her in.

'But why should I?' she asked. 'I'm very well as I am.'

'Gracious,' said the folks. 'Are you not afraid to be on your own in that lonesome place? Think of all the wild beasts around,' they said.

'Well,' said the girl. 'You know there are no wild beasts in the forest except perhaps a deer or two or a hare or fox.'

But the folk were worried for her, for you never could tell. The forest was big and dark, anybody could be there and there might be worse things than wild beasts.

'What?' she asked.

They looked to the left and they looked to the right and they put their heads close to her ear and said, 'The wee people.'

'Oh,' she said. 'Goblins and ghosties and such like old wives' tales to scare the children?'

They were horrified. Did she not believe in the wee folk? Well she wouldn't say yes and she wouldn't say no to that. But what she did say was that if there were any of them why she didn't mind them at all. So they gave up talking to her about it but what they said to each other was that she was very brave for a girl. And that is how it came about that she was a girl who couldn't be frightened.

The strange thing was that it was true. With her dog and her cat she was able to keep the hares from the garden and foxes from her hens. And if a bear had come to rob her bee hive (though there were none in the forest) she'd just have twisted his ear and swatted him back to the forest with the flat of her hand to his backside. As for the fairies, well if there were any about let them keep to their ways and she'd keep to hers.

True, she seldom saw money from one year's end to the other but the things from her little farm that she had over what she needed for her own use she could trade in at the shop in the village for whatever she couldn't raise or make for herself. So what good would money be to her the way things were? And being contented she was happy as the day is long.

Then one day one of the lads in the village looked at her and saw that she was the prettiest girl in all the countryside. Then, having taken one look, he took another and saw that she had come of an age when she might well think of getting married. He went and told a friend or two and those took the word of it to one or two more, and in no time all the lads for miles around were clustered at her gate like bees in a storm all hoping that she would choose one of them. All but William the weaver's son who had a croft on the hillside. He knew that she was beautiful and old enough to be married but he chose to bide his time and climbed up to his croft to tend his sheep. Little good came to those who stayed to woo her for she wouldn't have any of them.

'Why should I?' she asked them. 'To protect her.' Well she hadn't had any trouble doing that for herself. Besides she had her dog. 'For money?' Well she didn't want or need. 'For love?' And she only laughed and said that when the lad she could fancy came along she'd give them her consideration. But for the present, she'd stay as she was.

So at last all the lads were so discouraged that they left her to look elsewhere which did not displease her at all. The lads who had given up trying to woo her told William the weaver's son that maybe he'd done well not to waste time on such a headstrong girl and besides it wasn't natural for a girl to be afraid of nothing. But all William said was, 'Oh, we'll see then,' and went on tending his sheep.

So days went by and weeks went by, then one evening the girl went to the meal bin to fetch herself some meal to make some bannocks for her supper. 'There now,' she said, 'when I fill the bowl the bin will be empty. There'll be no oatmeal for porridge in the morning.' So she decided that after supper she'd take a sack of oats to have it ground at Hughie the miller's mill. So after supper she filled a sack with oats and set off for the mill. When she got to the mill she discovered that the miller and his family were away visiting friends. She decided to go further, to Lachie's mill in the next village. By now it was very dark but as she neared the mill she saw a light so she went and knocked on the door. The miller came to the door and stood there staring at her.

'I've brought you a bag of oats to be ground at the mill,' said the girl. And when the miller said nothing she apologized for visiting so late explaining that she hadn't any meal left in the house.

'I'll grind no oats tonight,' said the miller. 'Come back tomorrow morning.' The girl became impatient but the miller was firm. 'I'll grind no meal tonight.'

'Well then give me the key to the mill and I'll grind the meal myself.'

'O man,' roared the miller. 'I'll not grind your meal nor give you the key for when anyone grinds in the mill at night a great ugly goblin comes up through the floor and steals the grain and beats him black and blue.'

'Hoots toots to your goblin,' shouted the girl. 'I'll grind my grain, goblin or no goblin. Miller, give me the key.'

So determined was she that the miller fetched the key but would not give it to her until he had called his wife and all in his house to witness that he was not to blame whatever happened to her.

Then she took the key and the miller's wife gave her a lantern so she could see to grind the meal. The girl entered the mill, opened the water into the race so the mill wheel began to turn. She poured the grain into the hopper and sat down while the grain went through. After the meal went through she let it pour into her sack and knotted the top.

And just then through the floor rose a great ugly goblin. He had a big black club in one hand and he stretched the other hand to grab her bag of meal.

'No, you don't!' shouted the girl. She snatched the club out of his hand and began to chase him. Now the goblin had met many men at the mill but never a woman. He didn't know what to do as she had his club. The girl came after the goblin and banged him over his head with the big black club. She chased him round and round the mill and sometimes she hit the goblin and sometimes she hit the wall making a great noise.

The miller slammed the house door and he and his wife and the entire household put their hands over their ears to shut out the terrible din.

And then the goblin came up alongside the hopper where the grain was poured down. The goblin was about to pick up a great beam by the hopper when the girl came up close and planted her foot in the middle of the goblin's back and gave a great shove. Into the hopper headfirst went the goblin and the girl turned the mill wheel on.

So there was the goblin between the millstones flying round and round and round and round. It didn't kill him, for nothing can kill a goblin but it hurt him awful bad.

'Let me out, let me out,' shrieked the goblin, and he shrieked so loud he lifted the roof right off the mill. 'Let me out,' screamed the goblin.

'Stay down there,' called the girl as she wiped her face and smoothed out her skirts. 'T'will do you good.'

'Let me out and I promise you I will never bother you no more.' So the girl shut off the water. The mill wheel stopped turning, the goblin stopped screaming and all was quiet. But the goblin didn't come up so the girl reached down and grabbed him by the scruff of his neck and drew him out of the hopper. The goblin said not a word but limped out through the door of the mill and never again was seen or heard of in those parts.

The girl took her sack and went to the miller's house, 'Here is your key and lantern. I've ground my meal and got rid of your goblin so now I am going home.'

In the village William the weaver's son heard about the bravery of the girl. 'Oh dear,' he said sadly. 'She'll never be needing me now; she can look after herself so well.' He started up the road very slowly one foot then the other. But when he came to where the road went into the forest he heard something that made the hairs on his head stand up and he began to run. It was the girl and she was screaming at the top of her voice.

It must be a robber, thought William, as he raced towards her farm. He came to the door and rushed in picking up a big club that lay by the gate as he ran. He threw the door open and took a stand ready to battle whoever was there, no matter how many. And then he stopped.

There was the girl standing on the table between the porridge bowl and the jug of milk, holding her skirt to her knees, screaming for help with her eyes tight shut. And playing around on the floor was a tiny brown mouse.

William set the club down and leaned against the doorpost. He let her scream a little longer then said, 'So you are the girl that is afraid of nothing.'

The girl opened her eyes and cried to him, 'William put the beastie out; the dog is in the woods and the cat off in the fields. And there's nobody here can save me except you.'

'Perhaps you need someone to care for you after all,' said William. So he took the broom from beside the door and brushed the mouse out of the house. Then he lifted the girl from the table, took her in his arms and kissed her. 'We'll be married on Sunday,' said William.

'Yes,' said the girl and she laid her head on his shoulder as if that was where it belonged.

So they got married and were happy together. Sometimes William teased her about the mouse when she got too bossy. All was well understood between them, so no wonder they lived happily together ever after.

This final story is very relevant in a world where the impact of global warming becomes stronger year after year. A Sioux story to help us think about how humans behave in the world and towards each other and the consequences of our behaviour.

Remaking the World

There was a world before this world but the people did not know how to behave or to act human. The Creating Power was not pleased with that earlier world. He said to himself, 'I will make a new world.' He lit his sacred pipe in the sacred manner and said to himself, 'I will sing three songs which will bring a heavy rain. Then I'll sing a fourth song and stamp four times on the earth and the earth will crack wide open. Water will come out of the cracks and cover all the land.' When he sang the first song it started to rain. When he sang the second it poured. When he sang the third, the rain-soaked rivers overflowed their beds. But when he sang the fourth song and stamped on the earth it split open in many places and water flowed from the cracks until it covered everything.

The Creating Power floated on the sacred pipe and in his huge pipe bag. He let himself be carried by waves and wind this way and that, drifting for a long time. At last the rain stopped and all the people and animals had drowned. Only Kangi the crow survived, though it had no place to rest and was very tired. Flying above the pipe he called, 'Grandfather, I must soon rest.' And three times the crow asked him to make a place for him to rest.

The Creating Power thought, 'It is time to unwrap the pipe and open the pipe bag.' The wrapping and pipe bag contained all manner of animals and birds, from which he selected four animals known for their ability to stay under water for a long time. First he sang a song and took the grebe bird out of the bag. He commanded the grebe to dive in the water and bring up a lump of mud. The grebe did dive but brought out nothing. 'I dived and I dived but I couldn't reach the bottom, I almost died,' said the grebe. 'The water is too deep.'

The Creating Power sang a second song and took the otter out of the bag. He ordered the otter to dive and bring up mud. But when the otter came to the surface, it brought nothing.

Taking the beaver out of the pipe's wrapping the Creating Power sang a third song. He commanded the beaver to go down deep below the water and bring up some mud. The beaver thrust itself into the water using its great tail to propel it downwards. It stayed under water longer than the others, but when it finally came up it too brought nothing.

At last the Creating Power sang the fourth song and took the turtle out of the bag. The turtle is very strong. It stands for long life and endurance and the power to survive. 'You must bring up the mud,' the Creating Power told the turtle. It drove into the water and stayed below so long that the other three animals shouted, 'The turtle is dead, it will never come up again.'

All the time the crow was flying around and begging for a place to alight.

After what seemed to be a lifetime the turtle broke the surface of the water and paddled to the Creating Power. 'I got to the bottom,' the turtle cried. 'I brought some earth.' And sure enough its feet and claws – even the space in the cracks in its side between the upper and lower shells – were filled with mud. Scooping the mud from the turtle's feet and sides the Creating Power began to sing. He sang all the while. He shaped the mud in his hands and spread it in the water to make a spot of dry land for himself. When he had sung the fourth song there was enough land for the Creating Power and the crow. 'Come down and rest,' said the Creating Power to the crow and the bird was glad to rest.

Then the Creating Power took from his bag two long wing feathers from the eagle. He waved them over his plot of land and commanded it to spread until it covered everything. Soon all the water was replaced by earth. Water without earth is not good, thought the Creating Power, but land without water is not good either. Feeling pity for the land he wept for the earth and the creatures he would put upon it and his tears became oceans, streams and lakes. That's better, he thought.

Out of his pipe bag the Creating Power took all kinds of animals, plants and birds and scattered them over the earth. When he stamped on the earth they all came alive.

From the earth the Creating Power formed the shapes of men and women. He used red earth and white earth, black earth and yellow earth, and made as many as he thought would do for a start. He stamped on the earth and the shapes came alive, each taking the colour of the earth from which it was made. The Creating Power gave all of them understanding and speech and told them what tribes they belonged to.

The Creating Power said to them, 'The first world I made was bad so I burned it up. The second world was bad too so I drowned it. This is the third world I have made. Look: I have created a rainbow for you as a sign there will be no more great flood. Whenever you see a rainbow you will know it has stopped raining.'

The Creating Power continued: 'Now, if you have learned how to behave like human beings and how to live in peace with each other and with the other living things – the two-legged, the four-legged, the many-legged, the fliers, the no legs, the green plants of this universe – then all will be well. But if you make this world bad and ugly then I will destroy this world too. It is up to you.'

Someday there might be a fourth world, the Creating Power thought.

Then he rested.

Picture books for children

1. Mick Inkpen (1995) *Nothing*. London: Hodder Children's Books.
    This book has long been a favourite of mine with children who feel lost in the world. It describes the process of being recreated. The book tells the story of a little creature left in an attic. It cannot even remember its own name. The family move house and eventually the toy creature is reunited with them. Grandpa then remembers that the battered toy was a cat called Little Toby. He is sewn and washed and mended by the family in time to be the favourite toy of the new baby. He has found out who he really is and where he belongs.

2. Lauren Child (2002) *That Pesky Rat*. London: Orchard Books.
    This book describes a rat's search to find someone to care for him. He speaks to his friends about what it is like to be the

pet of their various owners. All have a good life but there are always disadvantages. Eventually Pesky Rat does find an owner, Mr Fortesque, who is so short-sighted that he thinks the rat is a cat and calls him Tiddles. Pesky Rat is happy and prepared to make the compromises necessary to be loved and wanted. I use it a lot with children living in a new or reconstituted family.

3. Lauren Child (2001) *I Am Not Sleepy and I Will Not Go to Bed*. London: Orchard Books.
    This is a story about Lola who is so active that she doesn't want to go to bed. Lola has numerous delaying tactics and Charlie her brother does all he can to appease her whims until finally she does go to bed and falls asleep leaving an exasperated Charlie to get himself to bed.

4. Lauren Child (2000) *I Will Not Ever Never Eat a Tomato*. London: Orchard Books.
    This is another story featuring Lola and Charlie. It is dinnertime and Charlie is expected to look after Lola and make sure she eats her food. Lola won't eat her vegetables. She is very fussy so Charlie tells her imaginary stories about the vegetables so that Lola eats them and eventually even chooses a tomato, saying it is a moonsquirter not a tomato.

5. Ian Whybrow and Tony Ross (2005) *Badness for Beginners*. London: HarperCollins.
    This is a funny story about a paradoxical family, the Wolf family, where the children are taught bad manners. However, Little Wolf finds it difficult to learn to misbehave. Some of their antics rebound when the parents trip over Little Wolf's mud pie and fall down Smellybreff's hole in the road. Funny and a helpful way to talk about behaviour and its consequences in a general way.

6. Colin and Jacqui Hawkins (1995) *School*. London: Picture Lions.
    This is a book which sums up school life in a humorous way. It describes types of kids, lessons and learning, nits and zits, mind your manners, nasty niffs, infections and afflictions, dangers and diseases. Then the dreaded teachers, school dinners and tortures. It is very funny and is a way to talk to

children about the perils of school life and connect it with their own experiences. It certainly reminded me of school days of long ago.

7.   Babette Cole (1996) *Dr Dog*. London: Red Fox.
     This is about the Gumboyle family and their dog, who is a doctor. It describes the family's somewhat disgusting ailments and physical problems from tonsillitis to worms and nits. Dr Dog himself finally succumbs to stress and takes a holiday away from the family but, alas, they follow him to his holiday hideaway. This is a good book for thinking and laughing about the physical self and describes ways of caring for the body to keep healthy.

8.   Mick Manning and Brita Granstrom (1997) *How Did I Begin?* London: Franklin Watts.
     This is a good book for younger children to introduce the facts of life from conception to the birth of a baby. The illustrations are attractive and full of charm and the text clear and developmentally appropriate for young children.

9.   Michael Rosen and Quentin Blake (2004) *Michael Rosen's Sad Book*. London: Walker Books.
     This is the moving account of the mourning process as experienced by Michael Rosen on the death of his son Eddie, who had appeared in many of Michael Rosen's books for children. It is painful to read but an honest and loving account. It is a shared experience for any child who has lost a member of their family or a close friend. I think it is an exceptional book.

10. Carl Norak and Mei Matsuoka (2007) *Tell Me a Story Mummy*. London: Macmillan Children's Books.
     This book is very soothing as it describes a farmyard where all the animals are asleep except Salsa the little goat. Salsa finally wakes her mummy who begins to tell her a story to help her get to sleep. But none of the stories are right for Salsa, so her mummy asks her what kind of story would send her to sleep. Salsa says she wants a sweet and gentle story. As Salsa describes the story she and her mummy fall asleep. The illustrations are quirky and calming and it makes a good bedtime read.

Books for young people

1. David Shrigley (2000) *Grip*. London: The Redstone Press.
   David Shrigley is a quirky artist and the humour in his
   drawings appeals to many young people. Though somewhat
   rude at times and dark, they can start a conversation, which
   can be an achievement with any adolescent. I like his drawing
   of faces with the text 'Faces in the Darkness. Some are your
   family.' *Grip* is a good example of his books and all his books
   of drawings have congruent texts. I often read them with
   disenchanted adolescents when we want a cynical laugh. It is a
   means of making a connection.

2. Ricky Gervais (2004) *Flanimals*. London: Faber and Faber.
   All the series of *Flanimals* are popular with children and young
   people. I often ask the young person to use the descriptions of
   the various flanimals to describe family members and it can be
   fun for the family to do this together. It causes much laughter
   and indignant denial.

3. Tim Burton (1997) *The Melancholy Death of Oyster Boy*.
   London: Faber and Faber.
   This is only for the uber-cool or morbidly inclined but the
   mordant humour and descriptions of gruesome children and
   outcasts struggling to be loved can strike a chord for some.
   The titles say it all. For example: Staring Girl; Stain Boy;
   Melonhead; Roy, the Toxic Boy. I write this as I look at my
   model of 'Junk Girl', a present from my daughter. We have the
   same twisted sense of humour.

4. Nicola Morgan (2005) *Blame My Brain*. London: Walker
   Books.
   This book describes for young people the new scientific
   research about the biological reasons for adolescent behaviour.
   The book defines what happens in the adolescent brain. The
   tests at the end of each chapter are really good fun and young
   people enjoy exploring whether, for example, they are risk
   takers and, if so, in what category they take risks.

Books for parents and professionals

1. Carolyn Webster-Stratton (2005) *The Incredible Years.* Seattle: Incredible Years.
    This is an excellent book for parents and professionals for dipping in and out to find ideas about managing children's behaviour. It is a guide for children aged 2–8 years, but it is helpful for young people who are struggling in the family.

2. Judy Dunn (2004) *Children's Friendships.* Oxford: Blackwell Publishing.
    This is an excellent book about children's friendships based on research in the UK and US. The book describes children's friendships at various ages and how parents can help over friendship difficulties. Her earlier book on young children's close relationships is also an informative read.

3. Taro Gomi (2003 and 2005) *The Doodle Book 1* and *The Doodle Book 2.* London: Thames and Hudson.
    These are books of doodles to complete and can be a way of attuning to children if adult and child play together. I do not always use the instructions which go with the doodles but just develop the drawings as the child and I see fit.

Art books

1. Ruth Thomson (2003) *A First Look at Art: Families* and *A First Look at Art: Places.* London: Chrysalis Children's Books.
    These two books help children to appreciate art but they include explorations of families and places that are pertinent for children and adults in thinking about their lives together. Each page is full of ideas about drawing and there are suggestions for activities that can be used by all family members.

2. Quentin Blake and John Cassidy (1999) *Drawing for the Artistically Undiscovered.* London: Scholastic.
    This is a fun book about drawing, a sketchbook full of suggestions and ideas to draw in the book. There are helpful ideas about drawing aspects of people – for example a page

on human anatomy in Quentin Blake style – and dogs and rabbits, etc. You get two pencils and a pen as well for drawing. It is a helpful way to think about identity and the physical self in the environment indirectly through drawing.

Soothing the adult with children's rhymes

1. Iona Opie (1988) *Tail Feathers from Mother Goose. The Opie Rhyme Book*. London: Walker Books.
    This book is still available. It is a book of rhymes and illustrations by a variety of artists. It is a soothing book with memories of childhood and after a difficult day can remind the adult of the pleasures of childhood games and rhymes. I like the dedication:

    > I am as I am
    > And so is a stone
    > And them as don't like me
    > Must leave me alone.

References

Ainsworth, M.D.S., Blehar, M.C., Waters, E. and Wall, S. (1978) *Patterns of Attachment: A Psychological Study of the Strange Situation.* Hillsdale, NJ: Lawrence Erlbaum.

American Psychiatric Association (APA) (1994) *Diagnostic and Statistical Manual of Mental Disorders,* 4th Edition. Washington, DC: American Psychiatric Association.

Anderson, H. and Goolishian, H. (1992) 'The Client is the Expert: A Not Knowing Approach to Therapy.' In S. McNamee and K.J. Gergen (eds) *Therapy as Social Construction.* London: Sage.

Anna Freud Centre (n.d.) *The Adoption and Attachment Represebtations Study.* London: Anna Freud Centre. Available at www.annafreudcentre.org/adoption.htm, accessed on 15 October 2007.

Aries, P. (1960) *Centuries of Childhood.* Reprinted 1986. Harmondsworth: Penguin.

Avery, G. and Briggs, J. (eds) (1989) *Children and their Books.* Oxford: Oxford University Press.

Bateson, G. (1972) *Steps to an Ecology of Mind.* First published 1955. New York, NY: Chandler.

Bergen, D. (2002) 'The role of pretend play in children's cognitive development.' *Early Childhood Research and Practice 4,* 1, 1–14.

Bowlby, J. (1969–80) *Attachment and Loss,* vols. 1–3. New York, NY: Basic Books.

Broks, P. (2003) *Into the Silent Land.* London: Atlantic Books.

Bruner, J. (1990) *Acts of Meaning.* Cambridge, MA: Harvard University Press.

Burr, V. and Butt, T. (2000) 'Psychological Distress and Postmodern Thought.' In D. Fee (ed.) *Pathology and the Postmodern.* London: Sage.

Cattanach, A. (1997) *Children's Stories in Play Therapy.* London: Jessica Kingsley Publishers.

ChildLine (2007) 'How to Beat Bullying.' Available at: www.childline.org.uk/extra/bullyingindex.asp, accessed on 9 July 2007.

Christensen, P. (2000) 'Childhood and Cultural Constitution of Vulnerable Bodies.' In A. Prout (ed.) *The Body, Childhood and Society.* London: Macmillan.

Corsaro, W. (1997) *The Sociology of Childhood.* Thousand Oaks, CA: Pine Forge Press.

Cowie, J. (2004) 'Challenging school bullying with peer support.' *Compass 17,* 1, 19–23.

Cunningham, H. (2006) *The Invention of Childhood.* London: BBC Books.

Dodge, K. (1983) 'Behavioural antecedents of peer social status.' *Child Development 54,* 1386–1399.

Dunn, J. (1993) *Young Children's Close Relationships.* London: Sage.

Eisen, M. and Goodman, G. (1998) 'Trauma, memory and suggestibility in children.' *Development and Psychopathology 10,* 717–738.

Engel, S. (1995) *The Stories Children Tell.* New York, NY: W.H. Freeman.

Field, T., Healy, B., Goldstein, S., Perry, S., Bendell, D., Schanberg, S., Zimmerman, E. and Kuhn, C. (1988) 'Infants of depressed mothers show "depressed" behaviour even with non depressed adults.' *Child Development 59*, 1569–1579.

Frayn, M. (2006) *The Human Touch.* London: Faber and Faber.

George, C., Kaplan, N. and Main, M. (1985) *The Berkeley Adult Atttachment Interview.* Unpublished protocol, University of California, Berkeley.

Gervais, R. (2004) *Flanimals.* London: Faber and Faber.

Goolishian, H. (1990) 'Family therapy: An evolving story.' *Contemporary Family Therapy 12*, 3, 173–180.

Greenspan, S. and Wieder, S. (1993) 'Regulation Disorders.' In Charles H. Zeanah Jr (ed.) *Handbook of Infant Mental Health.* New York, NY: Guilford Press.

Grotpeter, J. and Crick, N. (1996) 'Relational aggression, overt aggression, and friendship.' *Child Development 67*, 2328–2338.

Harris, P. (1994) 'The child's understanding of emotion: Developmental change and the family environment.' *Journal of Child Psychology and Psychiatry 35*, 1, 3–28.

Harris, P. (2000) *The Work of the Imagination.* Oxford: Blackwell Publishers.

Hendrick, H. (1990) 'Constructions and Reconstructions of British Childhood.' In A. James and B. Prout (eds) *Constructing and Reconstructing Childhood.* Basingstoke: Falmer Press.

Huizinga, J. (1949) *Homo Ludens.* London: Routledge and Kegan Paul.

Johnson, J., Christie, J. and Yawkey, T. (1999) *Play and Early Childhood Development*, 2nd edn. New York: Longman.

Joseph Rowntree Foundation (2000) 'Barriers to Change in the Social Care of Children.' Available at: www.jrf.org.uk/Knowledge/findings/socialcare/ 380.asp, accessed on12 July 2007.

Kidscape (2007) 'Top 10 Frustrations of Parents of Bullied Children.' Available at: www.kidscape.org.uk/parents/top10frustrations.html, accessed on 5 July 2007.

Laursen, B., Hartup, W. and Keplas, A. (1996) 'Towards understanding peer culture.' *Merrill-Palmer Quarterly 42*, 76–102.

Lewis, V. and Boucher, J. (1988) 'Spontaneous uninstructed and elicited play in relatively able autistic children.' *British Journal of Developmental Psychology 6*, 4, 325–339.

Libby, S., Powell, S., Messer, D. and Jordan, R. (1997) 'Imitation of pretend play acts by children with autism and Downs syndrome.' *Journal of Autism and Developmental Disorders 27*, 4, 365–383.

Main, M. (1991) 'Metacognitive Knowledge, Metacognitive Monitoring, and Singular (Coherent) vs. Multiple (Incoherent) Model of Attachment: Findings and Directions for Future Research.' In C.M. Parkes, J. Stevenson-Hinde and P. Marris (eds) *Attachment Across the Life Cycle.* London: Routledge.

McCartney, J. (2007) 'The Baby of All Battles.' *Sunday Telegraph*, 1 April.

Newcomb, A. and Bukowski, W. (1984) 'A longitudinal study of the utility of social preference and social impact sociometric classification schemes.' *Child Development 55*, 1434–1447.

Newcomb, A., Bukowski, W. and Pattee, L. (1993) 'Children's peer relations: A meta-analytic review of popular rejected, neglected, controversial and average sociometric status.' *Psychological Bulletin 113*, 99–128.

Novosyolova, S. (1991) 'Zur Genese des sujet-Rollenspiels-dargestellt auf der Grundlage der Theorie der Tatigkeit.' In H. Retter (ed.) *Kinderspiel und Kindheit in Ost und West.* Bad Heilbrunn: Klinkhardt.

Olweus, D. and Limber, S. (1998) *Bullying Prevention Programme.* Boulder: University of Colorado.

Parker, J. and Gottman, J. (1989) 'Social and Emotional Development in a Relational Context: Friendship Interaction from Early Childhood to Adolescence.' In T. Berndt and G. Ladd (eds) *Peer Relations in Child Development.* New York, NY: Wiley.

Richert, R., Lillard, A. and Vaish, A. (2002) 'Toddlers' Behaviours During Maternal Pretense Episodes.' Poster presented at the International Conference on Infant Studies, Toronto, Canada.

Rubin, K.H., Coplan, R., Chen, X., Buskirk, A.A., Wojslawowicz, J.C. (2005) 'Peer Relationships in Childhood.' In M.A. Bornsteing and M.E. Lamb (eds) *Developmental Psychology: An Advanced Textbook,* 5th edn. Hillsdale, NJ: Erlbaum.

The School of Manners (1983) London: The Oregon Press.

Schore, A. (2003) *Affect Regulation and the Repair of the Self.* New York, NY: W.W. Norton.

Sherbourne, V. (1990) *Developmental Movement for Children.* Cambridge: Cambridge University Press.

Shrigley, D. (2003) *Who I Am and What I Want.* London: Redstone Press.

Simpson, B. (2000) 'The Body as a Site of Contestation in School.' In A. Prout (ed.) *The Body, Childhood and Society.* London: Macmillan.

Social Services Inspectorate Report (1997) *When Leaving Home is also Leaving Care: An Inspection of Services for Young People Leaving Care.* London: Department of Health.

Sroufe, L. (1995) *Emotional Development: The Organisation of Emotional Life in the Early Years.* New York, NY: Cambridge University Press.

Stagnitti, K. and Jellie, L. (1998) *Play to Learn.* West Brunswick, Victoria: Co-ordinates Publications.

Steele, H. (2002) 'State of the art: Attachment theory.' *The Psychologist 15,* 10, 518–522.

Stern, D. (1985) *The Interpersonal World of the Infant.* New York, NY: Basic Books.

Storr, C. (1958) *Marianne Dreams.* London: Faber and Faber.

UNICEF (2007) 'An Overview of Child Well-being in Rich Countries.' *Innocenti Report Card. 7.* Florence: Innocenti Research Centre. Available at: www.unicef-icdc.org/publications/pdf/rc7_eng.pdf

Vandenberg, B. (1986) 'Play, Myth and Hope.' In R. van der Kooij and J. Hellendoorn (eds) *Play, Play Therapy, Play Research.* Lisse: Swets and Zerlinger BV.

Van der Kolk, B. (1994) 'The body keeps the score.' *Harvard Review of Psychiatry 1,* 5, 253–265.

Van der Kolk, B., Van der Hart, O. and Marmar, C. (1996) 'Dissociation and Information Processing in Posttraumatic Stress Disorder.' In B. Van der Kolk (ed.) *Traumatic Stress.* New York, NY: The Guilford Press.

Vygotsky, L. (1978) *Mind in Society.* Cambridge, MA: Harvard University Press.

Warner, M. (1994) *Managing Monsters.* London: Vintage UK.

White, M. (2005) 'An Outline of Narrative Therapy.' Available at: www.massey.ac.nz/~alock/virtual/white.htm, accessed on 12 July 2007.

White, M. and Epston, D. (1990) *Narrative Means to Therapeutic Ends.* New York, NY: W.W. Norton.

Wiedemann, T. (1989) *Adults and Children in the Roman Empire.* London: Routledge.

Subject Index

Author Index

Lightning Source UK Ltd.
Milton Keynes UK
30 October 2010

162122UK00002B/5/P